Alzheimer's Early Stages

. . . .

Selected Reviews

" … an Alzheimer's classic to be sure. A must-have for the well-read persons interested in Alzheimer's disease."
— American Journal of Alzheimer's Disease

"Kuhn guides families in developing a philosophy of care, offering clear and current information on the nature of the illness…this is a much needed addition to the Alzheimer's literature."
— Library Journal

"*Alzheimer's Early Stages* is practical, authoritative, and written with a clarity that will be appreciated by the general reader."
— Reviewer's Bookwatch

"Daniel Kuhn…writes with calm authority about a disease that is legendary for creating fear, confusion, and loneliness. His approach is realistic but reassuring."
— The Birmingham News

" … (the author's) hands-on experience with and empathy for persons with dementia and their caregivers jump off the page in this impressive new book."
— Early Alzheimers: A Forum for Early Stage Dementia Care

" …does a sensitive and comprehensive job of addressing the medical, emotional, and practical concerns inherent in the early stages…. It is a valuable addition to the Alzheimer's literature and Mr. Kuhn is to be commended for this very worthwhile contribution."
— Perspectives: A Newsletter for Individuals Diagnosed with Alzheimer's Disease

"Daniel Kuhn's book is a welcome addition to the caregiver literature."
— Family Caregiver Alliance *newsletter*

" ... highly recommended as a state-of-the-art review on managing the disease and the people who care for them. No social worker's library should be without Kuhn's book."

— Journal of Social Work in Long Term Care

"Dan Kuhn has been listening to persons with AD and their families throughout his many years of practice and has put this understanding to good use in this book. Social workers will be pleased to have this excellent resource to recommend to their clients."

— Social Work AGEnda, Newsletter of the Association for Gerontology in Socal Work

What others are saying about this book...

"I would highly recommend this book to our families that are dealing with a new diagnosis in an early stage patient, and also to professional caregivers working with patients in the early stages."

— Daniel L. Paris, Massachusetts General Hospital, Memory Disorders Clinic

"Dan Kuhn helps fill a void in the literature by offering families a wealth of insightful and practical information about early-stage Alzheimer's disease, something that too many families and patients have suffered through alone."

— Mark A. Sager, M.D., Professor of Medicine, University of Wisconsin Medical School and Director, Wisconsin Alzheimer's Institute

"Alzheimer's Early Stages presents thoughtful, practical guidance for caregivers based on up-to-date scientific studies. The information provided is of the highest quality, and the guidance offered is thoroughly wise."

— Stephen G. Post, Ph.D., Professor of Bioethics, School of Medicine, Case Western Reserve University and author of The Moral Challenge of Alzheimer's Disease

"This well-written, thoughtful and informative book should be on the shelf of every health-care provider and should also be recommended to those who are beginning their journey of caring for a person with Alzheimer's disease. Dan Kuhn is a knowledgeable, kind, and practical man, and readers will reap the benefits of his wisdom and sensitivity."

— Mary S. Mittelman, DrPH, and Cynthia Epstein, MSW, New York University School of Medicine's Alzheimer's Disease Center and coauthors of Counseling the Alzheimer's Caregiver: A Resource for Health Care Professionals

"*Alzheimer's Early Stages* is a must-have book for anyone diagnosed with the disease and his or her family members. Thoughtful, informative, and wide-ranging, it answers the questions any of us have when facing this challenging disease."

— *David Troxel, MPH, coauthor of* The Best Friends Approach to Alzheimer's Disease *and CEO, California Central Coast Alzheimer's Association*

"With the plethora of publications on Alzheimer's disease, few capture the biopsychosocial aspects of the illness with the clarity and understanding of Dan Kuhn. This book combines clinical experience and acumen with knowledge of the research and science. With a crisp writing style and logical presentations, this book is recommended for all clinicians working with those with Alzheimer's disease and their families."

— *Sanford Finkel, M.D., Professor of Clinical Psychiatry, University of Chicago Medical School and Director, Leonard Schanfield Research Institute, Council for Jewish Elderly*

"This book will be of interest to those who care for people with Alzheimer's disease: families, friends, and others who provide direct care. It's chock full of information and advice for caregivers and professionals in the field of eldercare. It provides compassionate support for anyone involved in the care of a person with dementia."

— *Mary Tellis-Nayak, RN, MSN, MPH, President, American College of Health Care Administrators*

"This book dispels the devastating image many people continue to hold of a person with Alzheimer's disease and promotes our understanding of the experience of the illness in the early stages. Both families and health-care professionals will benefit greatly from not only reading it, but using it as a resource and guide. It is both practical and wise."

— *Darby Morhardt, MSW, Director of Education, Northwestern University School of Medicine's Cognitive Neurology & Alzheimer's Disease Center*

"Dan Kuhn offers thoughtful readers whose lives are touched by Alzheimer's disease an excellent resource for information about the disease process itself, with a particularly fine section on the lived experience, ways to plan for and enhance daily life as well as essential information about caring for the self."

— *Carol Bowlby Sifton, BA BScOT ODH, Editor,* Alzheimer's Care Quarterly

DEDICATION

IN MEMORY OF ALBERT KUHN, GLADYS CURTIS, AND TO
ALL OTHERS WHO LIVE IN THE SHADOW OF
ALZHEIMER'S DISEASE AND RELATED DEMENTIAS.

. . . .

IMPORTANT NOTE

. . . .

Ordering

Trade bookstores in the U.S. and Canada please contact:

Publishers Group West
1700 Fourth Street, Berkeley CA 94710
Phone: (800) 788-3123   Fax: (510) 528-3444

Hunter House books are available at bulk discounts for textbook course adoptions;
to qualifying community, health-care, and government organizations; and for special promotions and fund-raising. For details please contact:

Special Sales Department
Hunter House Inc., PO Box 2914, Alameda CA 94501-0914
Phone: (510) 865-5282   Fax: (510) 865-4295
E-mail: ordering@hunterhouse.com

Individuals can order our books from most bookstores, by calling **(800) 266-5592,**
or from our website at **www.hunterhouse.com**

Alzheimer's Early Stages

Second Edition

FIRST STEPS FOR FAMILIES, FRIENDS AND CARE-GIVERS

Daniel Kuhn, MSW

Hunter House PUBLISHERS

Hunter House Inc., Publishers
PO Box 2914
Alameda CA 94501-0914

Grateful acknowledgment is made for permission to reprint excerpts from the following works: *My Journey into Alzheimer's Disease* by Robert Davis, Wheaton, IL: Tyndale House Publishers, 1989; *Living in the Labyrinth* by Diana Friel McGowin, Forest Knolls, CA: Elder Books, 1994; *Show Me the Way to Go Home* by Larry Rose, Forest Knolls, CA: Elder Books, 1995; *Who Will I Be When I Die?* by Christine Boden, East Melbourne, Australia: HarperCollins Publishers, 1998; *Partial View: An Alzheimer's Journal* by Cary Smith Henderson, Ruth D. Henderson, and Jackie H. Main, Dallas, TX: Southern Methodist University Press, 1998. *All rights reserved.*

Library of Congress Cataloging-in-Publication Data

Kuhn, Daniel.
Alzheimer's early stages : first steps for families, friends and caregivers / Daniel Kuhn.
p. cm.
Includes bibliographical references and index.
ISBN 0-89793-397-4 (pbk. : alk. paper) — ISBN 0-89793-398-2 (cloth : alk. paper)
1. Alzheimer's disease—Popular works. 2. Caregivers. I. Title.
RC523.2 .K838 2003
616.8'31—dc21   2002151932

Project Credits

Cover Design: Jil Weil
Book Production: Hunter House
Copy Editor: Rachel E. Bernstein
Proofreader: John David Marion
Indexer: Nancy D. Peterson
Acquisitions Editor: Jeanne Brondino
Editor: Alexandra Mummery
Editorial Assistant: Caroline Knapp

Publicity Coordinator: Earlita Chenault
Sales & Marketing Coordinator:
Jo Anne Retzlaff
Customer Service Manager:
Christina Sverdrup
Order Fulfillment: Lakdhon Lama
Administrator: Theresa Nelson
Computer Support: Peter Eichelberger

Publisher: Kiran S. Rana

Printed and Bound by Transcontinental Printing, Canada

9 8 7 6 5 4   Second Edition   04 05 06 07

Contents

. . . .

Foreword

. . . .

For over twenty-five hundred years, people have recognized that old age can be accompanied by the loss of memory and other cognitive abilities. However, Alzheimer's disease and other chronic conditions of aging have been considered a public health problem for only the past quarter century. This is mainly the result of the remarkable increase in life expectancy that has been achieved during the past century. Fewer people are dying young and infant mortality is lower; we have better sanitation, immunizations, antibiotics; and most recently, there has been a reduction in mortality from heart disease, stroke, and cancer. The demographic trends became obvious in the United States in recent decades, when the elderly population was growing rapidly and the number of people with age-related diseases was increasing markedly. This "graying of America" will continue well into the twenty-first century. The recognition of these demographic changes led to the founding of the National Institute on Aging in 1976, and the funding of the first Alzheimer's disease research centers in the United States in 1985.

But even with this increased attention to the problem, only a small fraction of the estimated five million Americans with Alzheimer's disease currently come to the attention of the health-care system. The vast majority are living at home, alone or with families, slowly developing memory problems, but not seeking help. In these cases a sort of conspiracy exists between the person with the disease, their family and friends, and their physician. There is a silent agreement not to talk about the memory problems until the disease has progressed to a more advanced stage, when the signs and symptoms cannot be concealed and the condition cannot be denied. Unfortunately, this conspiracy results in the loss of precious time that could have been used to avoid crises, plan for the future, involve the person with the disease in decision making, and treat the signs and symptoms of the illness.

Why is there so much reticence about recognizing, acknowledging, and confronting Alzheimer's disease in an open and forthright manner? The answer is complicated, but this reticence is partly due to fear. For years, Alzheimer's disease has been dramatized as a disease that steals the mind, destroys the ability to recognize family and friends, leads to an inability to control bodily functions, changes personality, and ultimately leads to institutionalization and death. Too often I have heard statements like "Mom can't have Alzheimer's disease—she still recognizes me!" However, Alzheimer's disease does not develop overnight. You do not wake up in the morning with Alzheimer's disease, as would be the case with a stroke or heart attack. Alzheimer's is an insidious disease. In the words of Daniel Kuhn, it "appears like an unwelcome stranger... [who] slowly and gradually makes his presence known." Furthermore, the disease is not necessarily a death sentence or a harbinger of a stark reality worse than death. A simple fact is that the vast majority of people with Alzheimer's disease are old, have a mild form of the disease, and die from something else before the disease progresses to more severe stages. People with mild, early-stage Alzheimer's far outnumber those with the later stages of the disease.

Now that the dramatic images of Alzheimer's disease in its end stages have captured the attention of scientists, laypeople, and politicians, it is time to think about how the disease begins. Alzheimer's disease has a beginning, not just an end; and as with all beginnings, one must take the first steps before one takes the last. The problems encountered early in the disease and the advice required then are very different from what is needed later in the disease. This book enlightens us about these early stages. Mr. Kuhn seeks to replace fear with knowledge, in the hope that knowledge will lead to empowerment. What does the disease look like and feel like when it first occurs? What types of problems are encountered first by the person with the disease, and by their family and friends? How can these problems be dealt with most effectively? This is the first book written mainly for the families and friends of people with early and mild Alzheimer's disease. This book is practical. It tells you what you can and should do, and in some cases, what you should not do. Like a good cookbook, it provides guidance and advice but leaves room for individuality and experimentation.

This book is also about reversing the dehumanization that unfortunately is now associated with Alzheimer's disease. Although the disease should be feared and respected, it is not a cause for embarrassment or shame. Alzheimer's is a disease of the brain. It is caused by the accumulation of abnormal proteins that lead eventually to the death of the brain cells responsible for memory and other cognitive abilities, behavior, and walking. It is not caused by poor behavior. This book will serve as a discussion tool to encourage open and frank discussions about mild Alzheimer's disease among patients and family members.

Dan Kuhn has been working with older people with Alzheimer's disease and other age-related conditions for thirty years. For over a dozen years he performed this valuable work at the Rush Alzheimer's Disease Center in Chicago, a large multidisciplinary center devoted to research, education, and patient care, supported by the Illinois Department of Public Health and the National Institute on Aging. He now continues this work at the Mather Institute on Aging, the applied research and education division of Mather LifeWays, a nonprofit organization devoted to promoting lifelong vitality among older people. This book reflects Dan's considerable experience, wisdom, and thoughtfulness. He has directly improved the lives of many people with Alzheimer's disease and their loved ones. It is with great pride that I see his knowledge shared with those who have not had the good fortune to work with him directly. I sincerely hope that through this book, Dan will be able to reach out and improve the lives of many more people with Alzheimer's disease, as well as the lives of their families and friends.

— David A. Bennett, M.D.

Director, Rush Alzheimer's Disease Center, Rush Presbyterian-
St. Luke's Medical Center, Chicago, February, 2003

Acknowledgments

· · · · · · · · · · ·

I am indebted to many people for their inspiration and help in writing this book. Heartfelt thanks to my former colleagues at the Rush Alzheimer's Disease Center in Chicago for their support, especially Anna Ortigara, Judy Jaglin, Jacob Fox, M.D., and David Bennett, M.D. I am grateful also to my current colleagues at Mather LifeWays in Evanston, Illinois, especially those working at the Mather Institute on Aging. I am forever grateful to the individuals and families who have courageously faced Alzheimer's disease and who have allowed me to share in their love and sorrow. I am a better person because of all of you.

Thanks also to many friends who provided helpful comments and encouragement in this endeavor. Special thanks to Carly Hellen, Dorothy Seman, and the late Tom Kitwood for sharing with me their vision of a better world for people with Alzheimer's disease.

My gratitude extends to the fine staff and volunteers at the national offices and local chapters of the Alzheimer's Association and the Alzheimer Society of Canada. I am also grateful for the efforts of the many dedicated professionals and volunteers at research centers who are working for a world without Alzheimer's disease. A special note of thanks to the hundreds of men and women participating in the Religious Orders Study and the Memory and Aging Project under the auspices of the Rush Alzheimer's Disease Center for their ongoing help unlocking the mysteries of Alzheimer's disease.

I also want to express deep appreciation for my companions in the Elmdale Share and Prayer Group, who have nurtured my faith, and for the Augustinian fathers, brothers, and seminarians who prepared my spiritual path. Thanks go, too, to my parents, Bill and Elaine Kuhn, for their help when I needed it most. Finally, love beyond words to my dear wife, Nancy, and our children, Curtis, Elizabeth, and Peter. May their children some day read about Alzheimer's disease in history books.

Introduction to the Second Edition

• • • • • • • • • • •

It has been less than four years since this book's first edition was
released, but the fast pace of research into the diagnosis, treatment, and prevention of Alzheimer's disease already dictates
an updated version. Unfortunately, there is still no cure or proven
means of prevention within reach. More drugs are now available
to treat symptoms of the disease and more drugs that promise to
be more effective than the current generation of drugs will certainly come to market in the coming years. Scientists are finding
ways to detect the disease in its very earliest stages. There is now
intense focus on diagnosing and treating people with "mild cognitive impairment," an intermediate stage between normal aging
and Alzheimer's disease. Thus, there is an urgent need for drugs
to stop or slow down the usual progression of the disease. Most
hopeful for the future is research into preventing the disease.

In recent years there has been remarkable growth in public
awareness about Alzheimer's disease. Due in part to the growing
numbers of people affected by the disease, there appears to be less
stigma now and more openness in bringing the disease to light in
private and public discussions. People in the early stages of the disease are speaking out for themselves in greater numbers than ever
before. When public figures like Ronald Reagan, Charlton Heston, and Ann Landers announce that they have been diagnosed
with Alzheimer's, they give courage to others to be more open as
well. Today, their family members and friends are also speaking
out in greater numbers and demanding more research and better
services.

Nevertheless, ignorance still prevails in most quarters today.
People with the disease are generally not diagnosed or treated

properly. Their families and friends are generally not getting the benefits of proper education, support, and services. Society has not yet come to terms with the costly nature of age-related health conditions such as Alzheimer's disease. A vastly improved system of long-term care will be demanded by members of the "baby boom" generation as they and their parents grow older. Glimmers of hope can be seen in the National Family Caregiver Support Program in the United States, which funds new and expanded services for families caring for older adults with disabilities.

It has been personally gratifying to know that many individuals and families were helped by the first edition of this book. This second edition contains a new chapter drawn from the experience of family members who attest to the fact that there is indeed life to be lived after a diagnosis of Alzheimer's disease. It is my fervent hope that this edition will guide you and help you live life to the fullest throughout the journey into Alzheimer's disease.

— Daniel Kuhn, MSW

February, 2003

Introduction to the First Edition: Why I Wrote this Book

· · · · · · · · · · · ·

This book is intended to serve as a beginning guide for family members and friends of people in the early stages of Alzheimer's disease. Although many fine books about Alzheimer's disease have been published, this is the first one written exclusively about its early stages. The latest medical information about the disease is explained, including possible causes as well as current and proposed treatments. Practical advice about coping with the disease now and help in planning for the future are also offered. My goal is to shed light on the common concerns of family members and friends who are newcomers to this troubling disease. If you have a relative or friend who has recently been diagnosed with Alzheimer's disease or is having difficulties with memory, thinking, language, and other brain functions, this book aims to help you deal with the challenges at hand.

Alzheimer's disease appears like an unwelcome stranger in the lives of everyone it visits. This stranger does not intrude suddenly into the lives of individuals and families but makes its presence known slowly and gradually. It helps to get to know this stranger sooner rather than later, because this disease not only robs the mind, it also forces dependency on others, especially close family and friends. Alzheimer's disease may last anywhere from three to twenty years, and becoming familiar with the challenges of its initial stages can help you to prevent or minimize crises later on. Although life often becomes stressful for family members and friends of those with the disease, it is possible to make the necessary adjustments successfully if you start early enough.

Alzheimer's is too often characterized only in the grimmest terms, and anyone who is just beginning to learn about the disease can get caught up in this doom and gloom. The media tend to stereotype those with the disease as helpless and requiring constant attention. People in the middle and late stages of the disease are seen as the norm, and the experiences of their relatives are often depicted melodramatically. Popular books on the disease often focus on its most trying symptoms, making only passing reference to the early stages. The advanced-care issues described in such books may be frightening and depressing for newcomers to the disease. These future challenges may have no relevance for a long time—if ever.

The beginning of Alzheimer's is a critical time to develop a philosophy of care and ways of coping that will promote a good quality of life both for the person with the disease and for family and friends. Once you are armed with the information and advice offered in this book, hope and self-confidence can replace worry and fear. Although optimism alone will not alter the course of the disease, it can influence a healthier adaptation. I have personally witnessed the positive effects on those who have adopted the old adage: "You cannot control the wind but you can adjust your sails."

A cure for the disease remains elusive, though much scientific progress has been made in recent years, and an increasing number of treatments and means of prevention are on the horizon. And although some stigma lingers in spite of growing public awareness, having the disease should not be a cause of shame or embarrassment. Former president Ronald Reagan's announcement in 1994 that he had been diagnosed with Alzheimer's gave courage to those living with the disease. At the same time, his disclosure raised questions about the nature of the disease, particularly the issues related to its beginnings.

Not long ago, Alzheimer's disease was hidden from public view. In the United States the enormity of the problem is just now dawning on us: Nearly five million Americans currently have the disease and this number is projected to triple by the year 2050. Unfortunately, because of lingering ignorance about the disease, most people living with it are not receiving the benefits of a proper diagnosis and treatment, and their loved ones are not receiving good information about coping effectively. The good news is that the Alzheimer's Association and similar organizations around the world are working diligently to increase public awareness, to promote research, and to provide services to affected individuals and families. Government-sponsored programs are also furthering these goals. Nevertheless, much more needs to be done. Given the projections for the future spread of the disease, we are truly in a race against time: Alzheimer's disease may well become the most pressing health problem of the baby boomers and their offspring.

As a social worker and director of education at two organizations devoted to Alzheimer's disease, I have been privileged to hear the hopes and fears of thousands of individuals with the disease, and those of their relatives and friends. In their unique ways, they have expressed their thoughts and feelings about coming to terms with this life-changing experience, and I have quoted many of them in these pages (their names have been changed to protect their privacy). These men and women have been my best teachers, and I am grateful to them for how much they have taught me about this disease, especially the importance of living one day at a time. An important lesson I have learned is that there is no single right way of coping. Therefore, this book is not a step-by-step guide to the "correct" or "best" way to deal with this disease. Rather, throughout this book I have both addressed general principles about coping strategies and offered some specific suggestions. Whenever possible, I have relied on the personal experiences of others to illustrate key points.

Many family members and friends who are newcomers to the disease have complained to me that there is little information or guidance readily available about the early stages of Alzheimer's disease. A few have admitted embarrassment that their concerns seem petty compared to the concerns of those dealing with the later stages. Although every stage of the disease is difficult, the early phases can actually be the most troublesome because of ignorance and misinformation. My goal in this book is to provide hope to those who feel puzzled, worried, frightened, or overwhelmed by the presence of this stranger in their lives. Perhaps some insights drawn from the collective wisdom of others can help you to meet the challenges you face now, and prepare you for the future. Although there is little chance of a miracle cure being discovered any time soon, with some planning you should be able to find the grace that will allow you to persevere in the midst of adversity.

HOW THIS BOOK IS ORGANIZED

The first part of this book mainly concerns the medical aspects of Alzheimer's disease. This knowledge about basic medical facts will help you to begin dealing with practical everyday issues. Although these chapters are full of facts about diagnosis and treatment, you should not be too concerned about absorbing all of the details right away. A medical understanding of Alzheimer's is useful, but the challenges to living posed by the disease are far more difficult to master. Science may ultimately provide some answers about the mysteries of this disease, but in the meantime, you need help with day-to-day concerns. The medical information in Part 1 provides a solid foundation for this. Part 2 addresses the emotional, social, legal, and financial effects of the disease on you, on your family and friends, and, above all, on your loved one with the disease. Understanding your changing roles and responsibilities in relation to the person with the disease is critical. Part 3 specifically addresses how to best take care of yourself as you care for your loved one with Alzheimer's disease. Achieving a balance between your needs and the needs of the person with the disease is key to coping successfully.

The epilogue lays out a broad agenda for change in public policy concerning research into and treatment of Alzheimer's disease. It also offers suggestions in the event that you and your loved ones wish to add your voices to the growing number of activists advocating for increased funding for improved services for everyone directly affected by the disease. Finally, there is an extensive resource section in three parts: a list of the Alzheimer's disease centers in the United States that are currently funded by the National Institute on Aging; books and videos that will help you learn more about the disease now and as it progresses; and a broad range of useful Internet sites.

Although this book offers you some direction, from time to time you will need to consult competent professionals for specific advice about medical, legal, and financial matters. Choose these professionals wisely; their expertise and experience may prove to be invaluable. Your local Alzheimer's Association chapter or area agency on aging should be able to refer you to professionals with a proven track record.

A final note about the title of this book: Although the book is primarily concerned with caring for people with Alzheimer's disease, the ideas presented here may well apply to individuals and families coping with a variety of other irreversible brain disorders. The term *early stages* refers to the fact that the disease is a process that unfolds over many years. My use of the word *stages* is an attempt to indicate that you will face different challenges along the continuum of the disease. Also, I have deliberately avoided using terms like *patient, victim,* or *sufferer* throughout the book, and instead refer to "people" with Alzheimer's disease. Maintaining one's humanity in the face of this dehumanizing disease is perhaps the greatest challenge for everyone involved. I have also avoided the term *caregiver* in describing family and friends who care for loved ones with the disease. You are first and foremost in a pre-existing relationship with a person who has a disabling condition. Your role in giving care is secondary to your role as a spouse, partner, daughter, son, in-law, friend, or similar close relationship. Your personal commitment, knowledge, skill, creativity, flexibility, resourcefulness, and faith will ultimately prove essential in meeting the many challenges that this disease presents to you now and in the future. I pray that this book can help you in taking the first steps.

PART I

What Is Alzheimer's Disease?

. . . .

.

.

.

CHAPTER 1

The Need for an Accurate Diagnosis

*It is evident that we are dealing
with a peculiar, little-known
disease process.*

Alois Alzheimer

A ging is a process of change. As we grow older, our bodies change in a variety of ways. Our hair may turn gray or start to thin. Our ears may lose their sensitivity to certain sounds. Our eyes may no longer see as well as they used to. Our skin wrinkles and our muscle tone diminishes. Physical functions in general start to slow down. Older men are at greater risk of developing prostate problems than they were earlier in life. Older women are at greater risk of developing osteoporosis. We have grown accustomed to the fact that most people over sixty-five years old eventually become frail. In other words, these changes occur naturally with advancing age. But should all such changes be considered normal just because they are common? Should we simply resign ourselves to living with the illnesses and disabilities associated with growing older? Most people facing the prospect of decline in old age would answer such questions with a resounding "No!"

In 1900, an American's average life span was forty-nine years, but now it has reached seventy-six. What accounts for this dramatic change? As a society we began to believe that many life-threatening diseases could be treated, cured, and prevented. Improvements in public health during the past century have altered our expectations. Lifestyle changes and medical breakthroughs have made longevity a reality for the average person in developed countries. In other words, there is no need today to think that disabling conditions associated with aging are "normal" just because they are commonplace.

WHAT IS NORMAL IN THE AGING BRAIN?

Forgetfulness is a universal human experience. For most of us, forgetting something represents nothing more than a temporary inconvenience, since usually the forgotten bits of information are trivial. Although advancing age typically brings about minor changes in memory, thinking, and other brain functions, most older people tend to compensate quite well for these changes. And although older people may generally be more forgetful than they were in their younger years, this forgetfulness usually does not interfere with the overall quality of their lives. This condition is referred to as "benign forgetfulness." It appears that although the majority of older people experience this difficulty to some degree, the scientific basis for this change late in life is not yet completely understood. Those remarkable older people who do not experience this common change are often referred to as being "sharp as a tack." Famous people who were healthy and productive into their nineties, such as the late entertainer George Burns and the conductor George Solti, come to mind. Strom Thurmond served in the U.S. Senate until age one hundred! Perhaps customary expectations of eventual decline should be replaced with new expectations of productivity and vibrancy in old age. By one definition, successful or healthy aging experienced by this small segment of the population may be considered normal. However, the common forgetfulness associated with aging may be more typical or "normal" in that the majority of older people experience this problem to a degree.

Although most people aged sixty-five years and older experience a slight decline in brain functions, less than 15 percent decline in significant ways. At first glance, age-related forgetfulness may appear similar to the forgetfulness associated with Alzheimer's disease (hereafter referred to as AD). Then what exactly is the difference between these two states, one considered a normal part of aging and the other a sign of disease? There is currently no one test that provides a clear answer to this basic question although tests are readily available that attempt to differentiate between the two. It is most likely that memory loss and impairment of other mental functions are part of a continuum between "normal" and "disease" and differences are merely a matter of degree. On the most basic level, however, there is a notable difference between memory loss that is merely annoying and memory loss that disrupts one's life. For example, it is trivial to forget what foods one ate at a restaurant last night, but it is a problem to forget that one ate at a restaurant at all. When memory problems become severe enough that someone cannot function independently, then this degree of forgetfulness is indeed not normal.

Older people may occasionally complain about forgetting names or misplacing things around the home. They may also notice these incidents occur with greater regularity as they age. These moments of absent-mindedness do not seriously affect one's lifestyle and may simply be an exaggeration of forgetfulness commonly experienced by everyone, regardless of age. Most of these people would perform very well on tests of memory and thinking if medically evaluated.

On the other hand, a person experiencing persistent forgetfulness but no other apparent difficulty with thinking may have a condition called "mild cognitive impairment."[1] This term, commonly referred to as "MCI," describes a gray area between the benign forgetfulness commonly experienced by older people and the more trying and chronic problems associated with AD or a related brain disorder. MCI is characterized by mild decline in memory and other brain functions such as concentration and orientation. Psychological tests are now capable of distinguishing such mild impairments both from "normal aging" and from AD. Most concerning is the fact that MCI often, but not always, represents the very earliest stages of AD. There is now solid evidence that the underlying biological processes that cause MCI are, in fact, the same processes that cause AD.[2] Many individuals with MCI remain stable and remain independent with little or no assistance from others. However, a majority progress over time into the early stages of AD. Figure 1.1 illustrates how MCI fits into the continuum noted above. People with MCI are now being enrolled in a variety of research studies to find ways of slowing down the typical progression into AD. Meanwhile, many physicians are treating people with MCI with the same drugs currently prescribed for AD. Understanding how and why such changes occur in the brain late in life has become the subject of intense scientific inquiry in recent years.

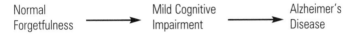

| Normal Forgetfulness | Mild Cognitive Impairment | Alzheimer's Disease |

Figure 1.1: A Continuum from Normal Forgetfulness to the Early Stages of Alzheimer's Disease

HOW ALZHEIMER'S DISEASE CHANGES THE BRAIN

Progressive severe loss of memory—routinely forgetting conversations or that one ate at a particular restaurant—and impaired thinking abilities are not a normal part of aging. Rather, such problems may be signs of a dementia—loss of brain functions due to an organic cause. *Dementia* is a generic term that includes a host of symptoms related to brain failure. Problems with concentrating, following directions, handling finances, and keeping track of conversations are all common symptoms of dementia. Just as we speak of many causes of conditions like heart failure, kidney failure, or liver failure, there are many possible causes of brain failure. And although there are dozens of causes of dementia, AD is by far the leading one.

The human brain is at the core of our existence, but we take its functions for granted until disease or trauma causes disability. Our brains enable us to think, remember, see, breathe, walk, talk, read, write, touch, taste, and perform countless other acts. Everyone's unique personality stems from a complex set of brain functions. Through the relatively new field of neuroscience, we are just beginning to understand the intricate workings of the brain and the disabling effects of brain diseases and injuries.

Essentially the brain is a high-powered communications network on a small scale—it weighs less than three and a half pounds. It has an amazing capacity to organize and execute complicated functions without any conscious effort on our part. The average human brain has an estimated one hundred billion nerve cells, or neurons, that normally work in harmony through a series of intricate chemical signals to store, process, and retrieve information. There are an estimated 15,000 potential connections, or synapses, for each of these one hundred billion cells.[3] Thus, the number of connections in the brain may total hundreds of trillions! Normal brain functions are threatened if a disease, such as AD, or injury disrupts cell-to-cell communication. AD destroys cells in the parts of the brain that control memory as well as other key functions such as reasoning and language, and when nerve cells in the brain die, they are not replaced.

When the brain is working properly, it is as if a huge symphony orchestra is simultaneously creating, playing, and recording a stream of masterpieces. If a member of the orchestra misses a note, then the music changes slightly but imperceptibly. As the faltering musician misses more notes, the change in the quality of the music is noticeable only to someone with a highly trained ear. Other members of the orchestra may play louder or work harder to compensate for the faulty or missing notes. If yet another member of the orchestra loses track of her part, the change in the music becomes obvious to others. Other musicians may be thrown off by the discord, and they too may misplay their parts. Soon, the most skilled and hard-working musicians may no longer be able to keep pace with the challenges of the diminished orchestra. Eventually the entire audience will start to be bothered by the strange sounds emanating from the once-perfect orchestra. This model of an orchestra that falters musician by musician until musical chaos ensues is a good analogy for the process of a dementia like AD.

AD unfolds over a period of many years. The slow damage to and death of nerve cells that accompanies the disease used to be visible only upon microscopic examination of certain regions of the brain. Recent advances in technology, however, now can detect such abnormal changes using brain scans. The disease typically occurs first in a thimble-sized area known as the hippocampus, believed to be the main recorder of new memories. It also attacks certain other areas, notably the cerebral cortex. AD is also characterized by reduced production of certain brain chemicals called neurotransmitters, which enable nerve cells to receive and send messages and help us to carry out innumerable functions, both intellectual and physical. When the brain no longer produces enough of these important chemicals, nerve cells can no longer communicate effectively, and they eventually deteriorate and die. Exactly how this process evolves in the brain is the subject of great speculation and controversy among researchers.

The nerve cells affected by AD are vital for memory and other so-called higher brain functions such as speaking, comprehending, reading, abstract thinking, and calculating. In particular, short-term memory, or the ability to remember recent events, is initially impaired by AD, but other brain functions may be affected at the same time. Moreover, nerve cells that control functions such as movement and vision may be well preserved. As a result, the physical appearance and bodily functions of a person with AD remain largely intact. The disease may be discerned only in the person's ability to remember, learn, and think.

In a sense, a person with AD loses the "glue" that enables new information to "stick" in the brain. This means, on the one hand, that if information is not sticking or being recorded properly, then new learning cannot take place as efficiently as it did in the past. On the other hand, information that is already firmly glued or recorded in the brain may continue to be retrieved from what is called long-term memory. This explains why someone with AD cannot remember a recent conversation but can reminisce in great detail about a childhood experience.

AD does not occur suddenly, as if a switch that's been in the "on" position is suddenly turned "off." Damage to the brain may be so subtle at first that no one, including the person with AD, may notice that it is happening. Nerve cell death and chemical deficiencies may continue over a period of many years before symptoms become evident. The slow and insidious onset is similar to that commonly seen among people with heart disease. Some people with AD appear to develop a mild form of the disease in which their symptoms may not worsen for five or even ten years. Indeed, they may develop other life-threatening conditions before the disease truly disables them. Other people with AD decline rapidly to the point of total disability within just a few years. Reasons for these different rates of decline are still not clear.

AD has probably been around ever since human beings first managed to extend life beyond six or more decades, although relatively few people in the West lived to an advanced age until the twentieth century. Over two thousand years ago, Plato commented that "a man under the influence of old age could not be responsible for his crimes." Writing in the second century, the Greek physician Galen theorized that a physical ailment might be responsible for the mental decline of some older persons. In centuries past, the symptoms now attributed to AD were referred to as insanity, senility, or hardening of the arteries. Then, in 1907, a German physician named Alois Alzheimer published the case of a woman who died at age fifty-one after her memory and other brain functions became progressively impaired over many years.[4] Upon her death, Dr. Alzheimer examined her brain under a microscope. He identified tiny abnormalities or lesions, now known as amyloid plaques and neurofibrillary tangles, throughout her gray matter. He attributed the impairments in her memory, thinking, language, and judgment to these physical changes throughout her brain. At that time, the symptoms that Dr. Alzheimer described were fairly common among older people. However, it was believed that these symptoms were a normal consequence of aging, and they were known as "senile dementia." After Dr. Alzheimer reported his findings to the medical community, the symptoms he described were classified as "pre-senile dementia of the Alzheimer's type," referring to the rare cases affecting middle-aged people.

Finally, in the 1960s scientists discovered a link between this unusual disease affecting a tiny number of middle-aged people and the common condition of "senility" observed among elderly people. Both age groups not only shared similar symptoms during their lifetime, they also exhibited the same pathologic abnormalities or lesions in the brain. It was at this time that AD gradually became a subject of intense scientific inquiry. The story of how AD originates in the brain and manifests in behavior is still being written nearly one hundred years after Dr. Alzheimer first described it. Yet even today basic questions about whether amyloid plaques and neurofibrillary tangles are causes or effects of the disease are not fully answered.

Research into most age-related conditions, including AD, is still in its infancy, despite the fact that the older population in developed countries is growing like never before. In fact, the age group older than eighty-five is the fastest-growing segment of American society. In the year 2000 this age group was thirty-one times larger than it was in 1900.[5] AD is now estimated to affect nearly five million Americans, the vast majority of whom are over sixty-five years old. As many as fourteen million Americans will have the disease by the year 2050 if means of prevention are not found.[6] The so-called "age wave" is forcing scientific investigations into all aspects of aging. After decades of scientific neglect, the "little-known disease process" named for Dr. Alzheimer is finally getting the attention it rightly deserves. Yet in spite of major advances in understanding AD over the past two decades, relatively little is known about its underlying causes, and as a result, it has been difficult to develop effective treatments. Means of prevention or a cure will remain elusive until answers to basic questions about the causes are discovered.

GETTING AN ACCURATE DIAGNOSIS

AD is by far the most common form of dementia, but there are many other types as well. Some can be reversed with proper treatment, but most, like AD, are irreversible. Table 1.1 lists some of the less common types of dementia that sometimes mimic AD.

The first purpose of a thorough medical evaluation is to distinguish between reversible and irreversible forms of brain failure. Receiving a proper diagnosis is the starting point for understanding troubling symptoms, causes, treatment, and prognosis.

Table 1.1: Other Reversible and Irreversible Dementias

Some Reversible Types	Some Irreversible Types
Metabolic disorders such as a thyroid gland problem or vitamin deficiency	Vascular or multi-infarct dementia
Infections in the blood or spinal fluid	Lewy body disease
Major depression	Frontal lobe dementias such as Pick's disease
Brain tumor	Huntington's disease
Intoxication due to drugs or alcohol	Creutzfeldt-Jakob disease

With most diseases, there are simple blood or urine tests that can help a physician to make a diagnosis. For example, a small blood sample can help a doctor readily detect if a person has diabetes. However, no single, simple test currently exists to detect AD, which partially explains why most people with the disease are never officially evaluated or diagnosed. Tests involving blood, urine, skin, eye pupils, sense of smell, and spinal fluid have been tested and thus far proven unreliable in identifying a diagnostic marker for AD. None of them has any practical value at this time. Researchers are making great strides to identify a quick and easy method of detecting the disease. Using a variety of brain imaging techniques such as MRI (Magnetic Resonance Imaging) and PET (Positive Emission Topography), researchers are aiming to perfect a method of detecting AD in its very earliest stages.[7] Such tests are currently quite expensive and are no more reliable than a physician who specializes in making the diagnosis.

A specific diagnostic test for AD would help doctors to distinguish quickly between AD and related disorders. It might also help to prompt early intervention, when the benefits of treatment are likely to be greatest. Such a test may be on the horizon and will receive much public attention should it become available. Yet the symptoms of AD manifest in such a classic pattern that even without a single test, it is possible for an experienced physician to make an accurate diagnosis in the vast majority of cases and to differentiate it from less common forms of dementia.

Perhaps the most important part of a diagnostic evaluation involves gathering information about the past and current symptoms. People showing signs of dementia may have varying degrees of insight into the nature and severity of their difficulties. Therefore, obtaining an accurate history about the symptoms from a knowledgeable informant is key to sorting out the medical facts. The observations of spouses, life partners, close relatives, and friends can be crucial in helping a physician to make an accurate diagnosis.

Most types of dementia are progressive and the manner in which symptoms unfold usually will support or rule out certain diagnoses. A process of eliminating other causes of dementia is the typical means of arriving at a probable diagnosis. This is done through blood tests to look for chemical excesses or deficiencies, and a brain scan to rule out a tumor, stroke, or other abnormality. These tests can be done on an outpatient basis, and most costs are covered by health insurance. Table 1.2 summarizes the tests used to detect and sort out the symptoms of dementia.

Table 1.2: Components of Diagnostic Testing

Commonly Used	Sometimes Used
History and physical exam	Psychological tests
Neurological exam	Spinal tap
Cognitive screening exam	Brain scan (PET or SPECT)
Blood tests	HIV blood test
Brain scan (CT or MRI)	Brain biopsy

In most cases, it is not difficult to make an accurate diagnosis of AD. However, this disease does not protect one from getting other age-related diseases. Thus, identifying AD when it coexists with another condition can be difficult. Unfortunately, because of the lack of a single foolproof test, some physicians overlook the disease or mistake it for a related condition. For example, a person who is severely depressed may be forgetful in ways similar to a person with AD. Many reversible forms of dementia such as major depression, pernicious anemia, brain tumors, hypothyroidism, infections, and nutritional deficiencies may mimic the symptoms of AD, and many medications can induce memory impairment and other symptoms associated with the disease. A careful evaluation can yield the correct diagnosis, since the symptoms found in most cases of AD conform to a typical pattern.

A physician will use a number of diagnostic tools to sort out the facts. First, rather simple mental-status tests enable a physician to assess memory, language, and organizational abilities, and screen for the presence of cognitive impairments. The most commonly used screening test is known as the "Mini-Mental State Exam" and involves a brief series of questions and tasks that identify the presence and severity of impairments.[8] Performance of everyday tasks, such as handling money or using a telephone, should also be explored through a separate interview with a reliable informant. If memory loss or any other brain impairments are revealed, additional tests should be done. These include a physical and neurological examination, blood tests, and a brain scan. Although such tests seldom show abnormalities, every possible explanation must be considered. In some cases, further laboratory tests, brain-imaging tests, and psychological tests may be needed to clarify a diagnosis. However, a limitation of psychological tests is that they are often geared to older people with average levels of education and intelligence, and may not be sensitive enough to detect subtle abnormalities among those with high levels of education and intelligence. In such cases, close family members and friends can corroborate whether there has been a decline in mental functioning. Therefore, detailed psychological tests may be useful, but are not essential in making a diagnosis of AD.

As already noted, recent improvements in brain imaging techniques have made it possible to see changes in the living brain due to AD. However, examination of brain tissue under a microscope is currently the only accepted method of absolutely confirming the presence of AD. If a biopsy is performed, in which a small piece of brain tissue is removed surgically, an expert looks for the tiny brain lesions (plaques and tangles) that would lead to a definitive diagnosis of AD. However, a brain biopsy is potentially dangerous and is very rarely done. The most common way of confirming a diagnosis of AD is through a brain autopsy—an examination done after death. However, as stated above, a reliable diagnosis can be made without an expensive brain scan, a biopsy, or an autopsy based on a close scrutiny of the individual's symptoms. Certain criteria have been established to help guide physicians in making this "probable" diagnosis: [9]

1. There must be a gradual and progressive worsening in short-term memory and in at least one other brain function such as orientation, language, judgment, and concentration.

2. These deficits must cause significant impairment in social and occupational functioning and represent a decline in the person's previous level of functioning.

3. Other medical conditions that otherwise could account for the progressive deficits must be ruled out.

With the help of these criteria, physicians experienced in assessing people with memory disorders such as AD are able to make an accurate clinical diagnosis in the majority of cases. In fact, the accuracy rate of diagnosis by experienced physicians is 85 percent or greater, as confirmed by autopsy.[10] The remaining cases are typically found to be other irreversible forms of dementia, such as vascular dementia due to tiny strokes alone or in combination with AD. The specific symptoms of these related dementias are occasionally difficult to differentiate from the far more common AD.

THE VALUE OF A DIAGNOSIS

All physicians are familiar with AD, but not all of them are comfortable making the diagnosis. Some see the lack of a single accurate test as an impediment. Others refrain from making the diagnosis because they may feel inadequate in treating the symptoms of the disease. Still others mistakenly attribute the symptoms simply to old age, as if serious decline with aging is inevitable. Since drugs for treating AD are relatively new, some physicians may not be familiar with their potential benefits. Also, current drug treatments are modestly effective at best. Many problems associated with AD are intertwined with the psychosocial issues of families caring for the person with the disease, and some physicians, mostly because of time constraints, do not get involved in these complicated matters. Unfortunately, health insurance does not adequately reimburse physicians for the time and effort to deal with this disease effectively. Even the most compassionate physician may not be able to address the array of challenges presented by AD.

Nevertheless, these considerations should not deter a physician from making a medical evaluation or from referring you and the person with symptoms to a specialist. He or she may need to be prompted to take the symptoms seriously, which means you may need to make a phone call to the physician's office in advance of a visit, or engage the physician directly in a discussion about your observations. The changes you are seeing are troubling, and by any standard, it's reasonable to request a medical explanation. Assertiveness may be required on your part to elicit the physician's cooperation in completing a thorough medical evaluation.

Other good reasons for getting a timely diagnosis are summarized in Table 1.3. If a physician cannot personally offer this measure of help, then he or she should refer you to others who can be of assistance.

Table 1.3: Reasons for Obtaining a Diagnosis

- To rule out reversible forms of dementia
- To provide a context and explanation for symptoms (see Chapter 2)
- To obtain appropriate medical treatment (see Chapter 4)
- To let you decide whether or not to enroll in research studies (see Chapter 4)
- To help you understand your changing roles and responsibilities (See Chapters 6 and 7)
- To ease communication among all concerned (see Chapter 8)
- To plan for the future (see Chapter 9)

The medical specialists most attuned to diagnosing AD are neurologists, psychiatrists, and geriatricians. Nevertheless, all physicians caring for older persons should be attentive to the warning signs of the disease and in most cases should be able to rule out reversible causes of dementia. Specialists should be consulted in all unusual cases, and if there is still uncertainty about the diagnosis after an expert opinion, a follow-up examination in six months or a year may clarify the situation, since AD involves a progressive worsening of symptoms. Specialized diagnostic clinics can be found at all of the AD centers in the United States funded by the National Institute on Aging (see Resources in the back). Many states also provide funding for other diagnostic centers. These centers and local chapters of the Alzheimer's Association in the United States or the Alzheimer Society in Canada can refer you to a specialty clinic or other known experts in your area.

DISCLOSING THE DIAGNOSIS

After tests have ruled out reversible causes of dementia and the established criteria for AD have been met, the physician should sensitively explain the test results, diagnosis, and treatment options to the individual who has been tested, you, and any others close to the situation. The physician should also address questions regarding the potential causes of AD and the progression of the disease, and give recommendations regarding educational and supportive services. Ample time should be available for questions and answers. For the sake of informing others unable to attend this important meeting, audiotaping or videotaping should be allowed. With permission of the person with AD, you can also request a copy of the medical records for later review and distribution to other interested parties.

Family members and friends sometimes worry about the reactions of the person being given the diagnosis of AD. It may be useful for the physician to speak with you first, but this is not the suggested option. A separate meeting does allow time for your immediate emotional reactions and a discussion of the way in which the diagnosis will be presented to the individual with the disease. A fear commonly expressed is that the news will be devastating and depressing to the individual with the disease. These negative expectations are understandable in light of the grim stereotypes about the disease. However, the diagnosis is usually received with little or no emotion and few if any questions. For the sake of unity in your relationship with the person with AD, therefore, it is better for everyone to meet at the same time with the physician so that the diagnosis and reactions can be shared.

The full implications of the diagnosis are seldom grasped by those with AD. Even those who are well aware of their symptoms ordinarily do not appear overwhelmed by the news. It seems that the ability to understand the magnitude of the situation may be blunted by the disease itself. Those with AD typically do not share the same perceptions of the disease as others close to them. In a sense, the disease is often accompanied by a cushion that softens its meaning for the affected person. Most people with AD already know that something is not right with their memory and thinking. Putting a label on their symptoms may make no difference to them. However, receiving the diagnosis may eliminate their need to cover up or to try to compensate for their difficulties.

Some people with AD ask a few basic questions but usually defer to their family for clarification or further information. Still others admit to a memory problem but dismiss it as nothing unusual for an aging person. Some feel relieved that their symptoms can be attributed to a disease instead of something that they have failed to control with their willpower. After being told his diagnosis, one man commented, "I knew something was not right, so I have been working hard for quite a while to cover up the problem. Perhaps now I don't have to be so careful if others know what's going on with me." [11] This view was also expressed by Ruth Janusak in a video about AD: "The fact that I have Alzheimer's is something I want everyone to know. I want people to be sincere in what they say to me and I want them to know that I'm not contagious!" [12]

Others are relieved because they can now discuss their difficulties openly for a change instead of feeling embarrassed by their need for help. They may want to plan out how to make the best use of their time before the disease disables them any further. Yet others may also wish to take part in a support group for persons with AD in order to obtain advice and information about coping with the disease. Appropriate reading materials suited to those with the disease are noted in the Resources. Many people with AD exhibit little or no desire to further discuss their diagnosis and its implications, and they should not be pressed to do so.

The physician may opt to avoid the term *Alzheimer's disease* out of respect for the expressed wishes of the family. Vague wording about the cause or causes of symptoms may be enough to satisfy everyone, but this approach should rarely be followed. Years ago, physicians and families were reluctant to tell individuals about a diagnosis of cancer. It is now recognized that this deceptive practice created more problems than it solved. Openness and honesty have now replaced the conspiracy of silence that once prevailed in relation to disclosing the diagnosis of cancer. The same principle should apply in relation to telling an individual about his or her diagnosis of AD.

Moreover, a central principle of medical ethics is each person's "right to know." Everyone has the legal right to access the private information contained in his or her medical records. Disclosing the diagnosis enables people with AD to participate fully in decisions about themselves both now and the future. For example, the diagnosis must be given if the person with AD is to make an informed choice about participating in research studies. A diagnosis helps the person with AD and others to make legal and financial plans in an atmosphere of openness and true dialogue. The benefits of telling the truth about the diagnosis invariably outweigh the perceived benefits of secrecy. Even though a family may wish to shade the truth or avoid it altogether for its own reasons, this approach should be challenged. Nevertheless, since the family ultimately must live with the consequences of the diagnosis, each family's unique preference regarding disclosure of the diagnosis must be respected.

Although the hallmark of AD is loss of recent memory, there are many other possible symptoms associated with the disease in its early stages. The next chapter focuses on the many symptoms that may be manifested in the early stages of Alzheimer's disease.

CHAPTER 2

Symptoms of the Early Stages of Alzheimer's Disease

*I have recently been told that I
am one of the millions of
Americans afflicted with
Alzheimer's disease.*

Ronald Reagan, 4 November 1994

Forgetfulness may be sporadic and seem insignificant in the early stages of AD, but it becomes more persistent over time. It may take months or years before you, as a close relative or friend of someone experiencing gradual memory loss, begin to notice any pattern. A particularly troubling incident or a series of minor incidents may trigger an appointment for a medical evaluation. Although persistent memory impairment is the key feature of AD, subtle changes in one or more brain functions such as language, orientation, perception, and judgment may also be evident in the early stages. In this chapter, I describe how the disease may develop in the everyday lives of people with AD.

The early stages of AD usually involve difficulty remembering recent episodes—such as forgetting an encounter with someone or losing or misplacing something. These instances gradually begin to disrupt one's customary lifestyle. The person with early-stage

AD may require regular reminders about tasks such as keeping appointments, cooking meals, or paying bills. At the same time, people with early-stage AD appear to think and behave normally much of the time, an appearance that is deceptive, since the progressive microscopic damage to their brains is creating a host of practical difficulties. There may be valiant efforts to hide or compensate for such difficulties, but eventually, others close to the situation sense that something is not quite right. As the disease slowly advances, the need for help becomes more apparent. Therefore, it is important to understand the usual signs and symptoms of the disease, as well as many unusual features that may be manifested.

WHAT IS RECENT MEMORY?

The type of memory affected by AD is generally called "recent memory." A person whose recent memory is impaired typically forgets events that took place within the past hour, day, or week. Entire episodes or fragments of an episode cannot be recalled because new learning does not occur or is disrupted. Recent memory is quite different from remote memory, which involves events, places, or people from the distant past and often remains intact in the early stages of the disease. For example, a person with AD may not be able to recall what she had for breakfast today but may well recall the details of a high school prom some sixty years earlier. The ability to perform personal-care tasks such as dressing and bathing usually remains intact too.

Physicians have made numerous attempts to categorize the different stages of AD, but these classifications have fallen short for one simple reason: There is great variability among affected people in how the disease is first manifested and progresses over time, although impairment of recent memory is the common feature.

BEGINNING SIGNS

What are commonly referred to as the early signs of AD do not actually mark the beginning of the disease but are the first *observ-*

able and persistent signs. Recent research studies have shown that changes in the brain probably occur for years before manifesting as symptoms. Most family members of a person with AD are able to recall unusual incidents that occurred months or years before a loved one was diagnosed. At the time they may have dismissed these signs as nothing more than eccentric behavior or as a normal part of the aging process. Only when a pattern emerges over time are these strange incidents put into the proper perspective. The case of former President Ronald Reagan is typical in this regard.

Although Mr. Reagan did not reveal that he had Alzheimer's disease until November 1994,[1] his memory was probably declining for many years before he was diagnosed. When asked if Mr. Reagan showed signs of the disease during his second term as president, which ended in January 1989, former White House physician Burton Lee remarked, "It was noticeable that there was something wrong there, but we figured it was just the natural aging process. Nancy was going to protect him and she did. She kept him further and further out of the flow."[2] Others in the White House dispute this statement, claiming that symptoms of Alzheimer's were not evident at the time.

Nevertheless, some people observed disconcerting changes in Mr. Reagan long before he announced he had the disease. Edmund Morris, Mr. Reagan's official biographer, provides numerous examples in *Dutch: A Memoir of Ronald Reagan*.[3] Independent counsel Lawrence Walsh notes that in July 1992, Mr. Reagan was unable to recall his long political relationship with adviser Michael Deaver or the resignation of national security adviser John Poindexter. Former senator Edmund Muskie expressed dismay at Mr. Reagan's forgetfulness as early as 1987 in relation to the investigation about the so called Iran-Contra scandal.[4] To outward appearances, Mr. Reagan carried out his public life without much difficulty and retained his image as "the Great Communicator" throughout his eight years as president and beyond. For example, by all accounts he delivered a rousing speech at the Republican National Convention in August 1992. Although Mr. Reagan still had the capacity to deliver a prepared speech, it is quite possible that he may not have recalled its details a short time later. Such inconsistencies and a slow progression of symptoms are fairly common in the early stages of AD.

The full story about the initial signs of Mr. Reagan's disease has not yet been told. However, it is safe to assume that his early symptoms began to make sense only after a pattern emerged and a diagnosis was made. In hindsight, little episodes of forgetfulness that meant nothing when they occurred now take on new meaning. This is the classic pattern of the disease in its early stages.

Since we have no single objective test for diagnosing AD, it is possible for even keen observers to fail to detect the disease in its early stages. The decline in memory often associated with aging confuses the situation. For example, allowances are made for an eighty-year-old person who is a bit forgetful because of the common belief that some degree of memory loss is to be expected at that advanced age. But if the same level of memory loss were observed in a fifty-year-old person, there would be cause for alarm. In other words, societal expectations often come into play in distinguishing between normal and abnormal forgetfulness.

In the time between when Mr. Reagan first showed signs of AD and his announcement that he was in the early stage of the disease, he probably compensated fairly well for his deficits. Furthermore, others probably helped to cover up his difficulties, especially his devoted wife, Nancy. People with AD naturally follow a pattern of compensating. After all, it is only human to want to avoid embarrassment and to be at one's best in everyday situations. The individual with early-stage AD may look physically fine and retain a wide range of abilities, effectively hiding any problems with memory and thinking.

Many people with AD are able to continue compensating for their symptoms, keeping them hidden from others, even their spouses, for months or years. They may deliberately avoid embarrassing situations that challenge their faulty memory. They may quietly retire from their jobs, for instance, after realizing that work demands are becoming too challenging. Once they retire, others may not readily notice their deficits because they no longer have the intellectual demands of a job. At home, they may gradually turn over certain responsibilities to others, such as balancing a checkbook, shopping for food, or preparing income taxes. They may avoid new and unfamiliar places and people, and rely on stock phrases and old memories in conversations instead of revealing their inability to keep track of new details. These are not usually deliberate attempts to cover up, but unconscious efforts to adapt to changes in memory and thinking. Often their spouses and others close to the situation unwittingly adapt to these changes and slowly assume a more active role in the relationship.

Loved ones usually notice the problem once the affected person becomes taxed beyond his or her mental abilities. While daily routines may not reveal much, stressful episodes may bring symptoms of the disease into the open. For example, the drastic change in lifestyle required as a result of a spouse's death is enough to uncover symptoms. In addition to the loss, the spouse can no longer help in taking care of the details of everyday life. In one case, a son describes how he first became aware that there was a serious problem with his mother after his father's sudden death: "I knew [M]om was slipping a bit, but Dad rarely complained. He gradually took over most of the household tasks. After he died, Mom seemed really confused. She not only missed him on an emotional level but on a very practical level too. I had no idea of how forgetful she was until he was gone."

Any significant change in the routine of an affected person may be sufficient to bring out the symptoms of AD. For example, when a person with AD goes on vacation, he or she may experience confusion and may even get lost. One woman traced her first awareness of her husband's AD to their trip to Europe:

First, he did not participate as usual in the planning of the vacation. He seemed anxious while packing his bags. He had trouble remembering the location of hotels as well as our itinerary. He seemed really out of sorts at times but then he would seem okay at other times. He was fine when we got back home, but later I began to notice little things that made me suspicious all over again.

AN EMERGING PATTERN

Abilities to store, prioritize, and recall new information are brain functions that slowly break down with the onset of AD. At first, family members usually write off these memory lapses as absent-mindedness or a lack of attention. Forgetfulness may be easily overlooked as part of the human experience. After all, there are so many minute details to remember that the brain naturally filters out trivia. However, these incidents eventually become part of a disturbing pattern, indicating AD.

In the early stages, the affected person may be able to remember certain trivial details while forgetting matters of great importance, or vice-versa. Loved ones may rationalize these memory lapses as random blips when, in fact, they may be the initial signs of the disease. In some cases, the person with AD is the first to notice the problem and to complain about changes in memory and thinking.

Forgetfulness in the early stages of AD may take a variety of forms. At first, it is mild and erratic. Those affected forget things more often than they did in the past. They may forget appointments, parts of conversations, or even entire conversations. Even when reminded, they may forget again just minutes later. They may even forget that they have forgotten! Or they may repeat the same statements or questions over and over. Their attempts to compensate by writing out reminders or by having others repeat instructions to them eventually prove inadequate as the problem worsens. They may forget about appointments. They may forget to pay bills or they may pay the same ones more than once. They may forget that they have food cooking on the stove and end up with burned meals. Learning and remembering new information becomes a real problem.

The person with AD typically has good and bad days or good and bad moments within a given day. He or she may remember some things and forget others within the same hour. Ann Davidson writes in her memoir about her husband with AD:

> Julian can't remember that his underpants are in the dresser, yet he usually remembers to come home on time. He doesn't

know the location of the wall plugs when he tries to vacuum, yet he knows how to go alone to the library. He's capable in some areas, impaired in others. His abilities fluctuate day-to-day, maddeningly inconsistent.[5]

Such ups and downs may prevent others from putting together the pieces of the puzzle.

There is also an enormous tendency to deny the reality that a loved one's growing problems may be due to an irreversible disease. Family members and friends may act as if no difficulties exist, or minimize their importance so that the situation ultimately resembles the proverbial "elephant in the living room" that everyone tries to ignore. Sometimes a crisis has to occur before others awaken to the fact that something is not right: the person gets lost while driving, utilities are cut off due to nonpayment of bills, a fire results from food forgotten on the stove. In some instances, it may take an "outsider" to recognize that seemingly disconnected incidents are part of a medical problem such as AD. It is like the pieces of a puzzle coming together. My interviews with family members and friends of people with AD illustrate these common themes: a pattern of memory loss in the person with AD coupled with puzzled reactions in close family and friends. The following excerpts are taken from conversations with family members who were asked to recount their initial awareness of a loved one's memory problem:

George described how he first became aware of his wife's memory problem about four years before her diagnosis of AD at age seventy-six:

She was having a problem with remembering names that I thought was excessive, even for an older person. I could not accept that this was simply the natural aging process. When she was interviewed by our family physician, he said there was no problem whatsoever and that she was perfectly normal in every aspect. In turn, I accepted the medical opinion and did nothing at all about it for quite some time.

Fred looked back to a year before his wife's diagnosis of AD at age sixty-two:

It seems like during the course of that year she was becoming constantly forgetful of things, like misplacing her glasses and car keys. Any time she needed something she would write and staple notes around her purse handle. Sometimes she would have fifteen or twenty notes stapled there. I really took notice when I looked for the pills that she was supposed to take every day for her thyroid condition. It turned out that the bottle had been empty for a couple of months. When I asked her if she had discontinued the pills, she said that she had just forgotten. Around the same time, she also stepped down from her position at work because she said it was getting to be too much for her worsening memory.

Because of a family history of the disease, Lucy explained that she became aware of signs of it in her mother about three years before she was diagnosed at age seventy-seven:

We noticed my mother started to forget little things. We've had experience with this before. My mother's sister succumbed to Alzheimer's and my mother's father also lived to the very late stage of Alzheimer's. The forgetfulness was becoming more commonplace—simple things like where she put things around the house. I noticed another classic sign in the repetitiveness. We also noticed a drastic change in her personality over the past year—she wasn't as outgoing or adventurous as she used to be. So we had her evaluated by a neurologist who confirmed what we had suspected from the start.

Robert recalled a particular event that triggered his awareness of his mother's loss of recent memory:

The first time I noticed a real problem was after her hysterectomy, when she was recovering in the hospital. They wanted to train her to get around and use the washroom at home. She was horrified that she couldn't remember what her bathroom looked like at home, but she remembered what the bathroom looked like in a house that she lived in when she grew up, maybe sixty years earlier. She could see the past very clearly in her mind, but she couldn't remember the present. She thought she was going crazy. That was when I figured out there was something up. I could see that her mind at that point was very fragile and that the sedation and other medications had set this off. She was never the same thereafter. I know I began to keep a closer eye on her after that hospitalization.

Mike lived a thousand miles away from his eighty-year-old widowed mother and saw her just twice a year. He reflected on her beginning symptoms, six months before her diagnosis:

On the phone she seemed just fine, but when I visited her she repeated questions quite often and reminisced about the past more than usual. I discovered that she had not paid a few of her bills, but she gave some excuse that led me to believe that it was a mere oversight. When these things were happening, I was not alarmed at first, but my suspicions grew over time.

Dorothy recalled the time she first noticed her mother's memory loss, about eighteen months before her diagnosis: "She would ask questions that I assumed she knew the answers to. She began to repeat herself, especially asking the same question that had been answered just a short time ago. I thought it was due to her aging."

Eleanor noted the change in her husband about five years before he was diagnosed at age eighty:

We were with a group of friends playing really simple card games, and he decided he did not want to play anymore. He said the games were stupid. Even then I suspected that he was just saying that because he could no longer remember the rules. He had always had an excellent memory but when he began to routinely forget appointments, I knew something was not right. My initial reaction was to insist that he make a greater effort to remember. I am afraid I put him through a miserable time.

As the above examples indicate, family members are usually puzzled by the difficulties that they notice in their loved one for some time before they realize that a disease may be in progress. Most people do not act on their feeling that something may be wrong, or they deny the severity of the problem. Waiting two or three years before seeking out a medical explanation is common.

Physicians, in turn, often do not detect the problem during a cursory examination or brief conversation. Consequently, most persons with early symptoms of AD do not receive a thorough assessment and diagnosis.

OTHER TROUBLING SYMPTOMS

Other symptoms may appear simultaneously with the impairment of recent memory, or they may develop over time. In most cases, although these other symptoms may be the first signs of AD, the central problem of memory loss doesn't lag far behind.[6] These difficulties are generally mild in the early stages but clearly represent a departure from the affected person's previous level of intellectual functioning or behavior. Table 2.1 summarizes common symptoms in the early stages of AD.

Table 2.1: Symptoms in the Early Stages of Alzheimer's Disease

Always present

▶ Impairment of recent memory

One or more sometimes present

▶ Difficulty with reasoning

▶ Disorientation

▶ Difficulty with language

▶ Poor concentration

▶ Difficulty with spatial relations

▶ Poor judgment

Noncognitive or behavioral changes

▶ Personality changes

▶ Delusional thinking

▶ Changes in sexuality

▶ Diminished coordination

▶ Diminished or lost sense of smell

ONE OR MORE SYMPTOMS SOMETIMES PRESENT

In addition to persistent loss of recent memory, one or more common symptoms of AD will sometimes be present in the early stages. These include occasional or regular difficulties with reasoning, orientation, language, concentration, spatial relations, and judgment. The appearance of such symptoms over time varies from person to person but all of them usually become prominent as the disease advances. At first, however, these difficulties tend to be mild in nature.

Difficulty with Reasoning

Reasoning, or the ability to think logically, is often the second area that is affected by AD. This impairment typically affects the person's ability to understand or solve practical problems. Like other symptoms in the early stages of AD, this symptom comes and goes. The affected person may become disconcerted if faced with a task involving a series of steps, such as handling money, doing calculations, cooking a meal, driving a car, or using household appliances and tools. Gloria explained that her husband had always been handy around the house but was stumped one day when faced with a relatively simple task:

> The first time I really began to notice there was a problem was one day when he tried to install a screen in the door. He stood there with the screen in his hand, looking at the frame and said to me, "I can't figure out how to do this." Then I began to reflect on other things that hadn't seemed right. I recalled that months earlier he had also said it was getting hard to balance the checkbook and had asked me to figure it out. He had always done the bills. These difficulties he was having were inconsistent, so I think we had been easing into things. When he said, "I can't do this" or "I can't figure that out," I realized that I wasn't just imagining things.

Disorientation

Confusion about time and space is fairly common in the early stages. The person with AD may get mixed up about directions and become lost or may not know the current day, month, or even year. Bill recounted the first sign of changes in his wife's ability to navigate their community:

> I noticed it in her driving at first. She had lived in our town all her life and always knew how to get around the area. One day she had to go to the bank and then to the insurance office. However, she had to come home after going to the bank because she didn't know how to get to the insurance company. She was also unable to keep track of her purse and was misplacing things. Her missing purse had become kind of a joke for the past four years. I think I just kind of grew accustomed to it, not necessarily thinking that it was Alzheimer's.

Letty Tennis writes in a newsletter about her warped sense of time:

> Time means nothing to me. I rarely know the day of the week or the date. This bothers me a lot, but we have worked it out. George just says, "You have an hour before we go, so start getting ready." Since time is not there for me, I nap in my chair sometimes and when I awake, I panic because I can't understand why I'm alone in the house—even though it's a work day for George. I'll dash around the house looking for George, or I'd have this awful feeling that I'm baby-sitting and can't find the children.[7]

Difficulty with Language

In the early stages of AD, affected people don't have as much difficulty with the *mechanics* of speech as they do with the *rules* of speech that make verbal communication effective. They might have trouble finding the right words or remembering names. Their ability to process information may be slowed, resulting in long pauses or lapses in concentration during conversation. The overall richness of their vocabulary may diminish and so may the ability to articulate thoughts and feelings and to comprehend the speech of others. (See Chapter 8 for more information about communication difficulties and for suggestions on dealing with them.) The first changes Winnie noticed in her husband were in his language ability:

> It was not so much his memory as his speech. Some of his sentences would be backwards. He would mix up the sequence of the words. I was getting frustrated and so I made an appointment with a neurologist, thinking that perhaps he had a mini-stroke or something. He was examined, but all the tests were normal at first. Another year passed before his doctor agreed that his memory problem had progressed and his coordination had started to diminish a bit. Only then did the doctor say he had Alzheimer's.

Poor Concentration

A person's ability to concentrate or to pay attention may diminish in the early stages of AD. This difficulty may manifest itself in reading with little or no comprehension or in being unable to follow a conversation. An individual may respond slower than usual to everyday situations. Richard noted that his wife often commented on her growing difficulty with conversations: "Sometimes during conversation, she would be talking and then there would be a lapse in conversation and she would say, 'Oops! The train left the track! What were we talking about?'"

Difficulty with Spatial Relations

The human eye depends on the brain to organize and interpret what is being seen. Judging distances and recognizing familiar people or objects are sometimes difficult for a person in the early stages of AD. In effect, the brain distorts visual images. This phenomenon, known as "agnosia," is an unusual first symptom in the early stages of AD.[8] The following stories by two spouses highlight how a difficulty with spatial relations heralds additional symptoms.

Frances recalled that her husband was the first to notice changes occurring in his depth perception:

He said he was tripping on stairs because he was having difficulty determining the space between them. It was as if the stairs were running together. He also complained that words appeared jumbled on printed pages. He would see things from afar and grossly misjudge their appearance. Of course, we thought it was his eyes at first, but the ophthalmologist said his eyes were fine. A short time later the memory problem emerged. Again, he was the first one to notice this too!

Don described his wife's early symptoms as difficulty with judging distances while driving, with other symptoms following:

About three years ago she was involved in a car accident on a road that was wide enough for eight trucks to go through, and yet she hit a parked car. I sensed that something wasn't normal when she had a couple more fender benders. After that, there wasn't really anything until last spring when I noticed she was forgetful, leaving purses, not taking messages, and she was not as neat with her appearance. Nothing drastic, but something was different. Also, people who didn't see her frequently would ask me what was wrong with her. They said she wasn't the same person—she wasn't outgoing or fluid with her speech and movement and thinking. I think it was the fact that other people were telling me that my wife had changed that made me aware of the fact that she was having these problems.

Poor Judgment

Making sound decisions depends on memory to an extent, but also requires logic and reasoning. Distortions in the thought process may lead a person with AD to make inappropriate decisions, even though she may believe she has made a correct choice. For example, one man in the early stages of AD impulsively bought an expensive new car, even though he could not afford it. In another case, a woman gave away most of her life savings to an unscrupulous neighbor. Another woman with AD turned up the thermostat in her home to eighty-five degrees, and the intense heat nearly killed her.

NONCOGNITIVE OR BEHAVIORAL CHANGES

In addition to the intellectual impairments described above, certain other symptoms may be present from time to time or regularly. These include a range of personality changes, delusions, and changes in sexuality, physical coordination, and the sense of smell. Again, not everyone with the disease has these symptoms. They tend to appear occasionally in the early stages and become more common in the later stages of the disease, but the frequency and severity of these symptoms vary from person to person.

Personality Changes

Personality changes are seldom dramatic in the early stages of AD. However, the affected person may not seem like his or her "old self" in some ways. The most notable change is usually diminished drive or lack of initiative. People who are normally active may become passive, assertive people may start deferring to others. People in the early stages of AD may show a lack of interest in people and activities that they previously enjoyed, such as family gatherings, social events, and hobbies. These changes in mood and behavior are often misinterpreted as a symptom of depression. Although symptoms of AD and depression can occur together, generally speaking a loss of initiative may be due solely to AD and may be unresponsive to treatment with antidepressants. Luke recounted the change in his wife after they had relocated to another state: "She had a complete change in her personality once we got there. She normally was outgoing and curious but she became a recluse. She wouldn't go anywhere without me. After a while, the confusion and memory problems set in."

Some people with AD may become self-centered and ignore the feelings of others. Such insensitivity may be offensive to others unless it is correctly interpreted as a sign of the disease. Judy initially worried that her marriage was falling apart because of the change in her husband's personality:

He no longer seemed interested in me, which was quite out of character for him. He became increasingly self-absorbed, to the point that I thought he didn't care about me, or anybody else for that matter. I was beginning to believe that our marriage was on the rocks for the first time in forty-nine years.

Some people with AD may become less inhibited in their speech and behavior. Someone who may have been calm and patient in the past may now seem short-tempered. Likewise, someone known to be passive and quiet may become opinionated and outspoken. Impulses previously held in check may no longer be fully controlled. For example, a daughter complained that her mother, who had AD, had always been "prim and proper" but had developed a pattern of expressing herself in an offensive way: "My mother never used foul language in the past, but now she is doing it freely with no hint of embarrassment. She can swear a blue streak, which can be very embarrassing. It's almost comical at times."

Sometimes people with AD may express a surprising degree of irritability or even outright aggression toward others, especially loved ones. Such disturbing behaviors typically stem from their feeling fatigued, overwhelmed, or frustrated. It is important for you to remember that verbal and physical outbursts are symptoms of the disease, and should not be interpreted as personal attacks. There is almost always an underlying cause that triggers these unpleasant occurrences. To the person with AD, hostile remarks and acts may be means of self-defense in response to situations that they perceive as threatening or to the confusion wrought by the disease. It may take some detective work on your part to figure out what triggers the antisocial behavior and how to minimize it or prevent it from happening again.

Delusional Thinking

Delusions refer to false, fixed beliefs. In AD, they usually take the form of allegations, such as of infidelity, financial exploitation, and similar personal offenses, against others close to the affected person. Delusional thinking is actually rare in the early stages of

AD, and it is typically coupled with the loss of recent memory.[9] Delusions may appear so irrational and out of character that they stir family members to seek a medical explanation. Peter noted that his wife became convinced that he was having an extramarital affair, in spite of all evidence to the contrary:

> She began to accuse me of infidelity—for the first time in fifty-two years of marriage! She claimed that whenever I left her alone I was seeing another woman. It was completely absurd, but she became wildly jealous and suspicious. All my efforts to reassure did not help. Only later did I understand this behavior as a symptom of her disease.

In another case, Joan's mother-in-law accused her of stealing some of her clothing. "It was preposterous to imagine that I would be interested in her clothes. She apparently misplaced some of her things and decided to blame me for some strange reason. She was convinced that I was at fault. Her continuing accusations really strained our relationship for a while."

Changes in Sexuality

Healthy sexuality depends on a variety of complex physical and psychological factors related to the brain, and there is some evidence that sexual dysfunction may be common in the early stages of AD.[10] Diminished sex drive is probably the biggest issue. Men may have difficulty attaining or maintaining an erection, while women may experience lack of vaginal lubrication. Whether these problems are related to disruption in brain pathways affecting sexual arousal or are a psychological reaction to other changes in the brain due to AD is not yet known. Maria described her husband's sexual difficulties: "He wanted to have sex, but he was unable to sustain an erection. After a while he gave up trying and I thought it was perhaps my fault. That was about the same time I first noticed his memory problem."

Sexual interest may actually sometimes increase in the early stages of the disease. Josephine explained the change in her husband's sex drive:

We had always enjoyed a close, loving relationship, but he became even more amorous after he suddenly retired. I later found out that his retirement was linked to his declining job performance. Shortly thereafter, I began to notice his problems with memory and thinking. Although his brain was failing, his sexual appetite was growing!

Because of embarrassment, many affected people unfortunately never address these sexual changes. Marriages may suffer over this sensitive matter, and spouses may retreat from each other or get into conflict. Partners of those with AD should recognize that changes in sexual functioning are not necessarily a sign of problems in the relationship. Rather, a diminished or heightened sex drive should be seen within the context of other symptoms associated with AD and should be discussed openly.

Diminished Coordination

Although mobility and other physical functions are typically unchanged in the early stages, sometimes a person with AD may walk cautiously or slower than usual, or have difficulty with getting up from a chair or out of bed. Most people with AD have minor difficulty with complex and fine motor functions involving eye-hand coordination and rapid hand movements,[11] which may be manifested in illegible handwriting or trouble using utensils or tools. This motor impairment may also get in the way of driving a car safely. How AD damages certain nerves and muscles while leaving most of the affected person's physical abilities intact is not yet fully understood.

Diminished or Lost Sense of Smell

There is also strong evidence that people with AD tend to lose their sense of smell.[12] This sensory deficit by itself is not indicative of the disease, since it can be caused by many other factors. Nevertheless, a lost sense of smell should be seen as another potential symptom of AD.

The early stages of AD are characterized primarily by loss of recent memory but may be accompanied by other symptoms. Loved ones may notice these subtle changes, but they are easy to miss. As the disease slowly advances, seemingly disconnected incidents of forgetfulness and other warning signs of brain dysfunction begin to form a troubling picture. You and others who are close to the person with AD should acknowledge disturbing changes and recognize that a medical problem is probably unfolding. A proper diagnosis, treatment, and planning are indicated for the sake of all concerned.

An experienced physician is the best person to sort out the various pieces of the puzzle and help you with the next steps. Your job at this juncture is to make sure that the physician knows about all of the symptoms and conducts a thorough evaluation.

Once a diagnosis has been made, there may be questions about the underlying cause or causes of the disease. Although researchers have identified no single culprit so far, I look at a number of possibilities in Chapter 3. Understanding the origins of AD clearly has implications for treatment and prevention, the topic of Chapter 4.

· · · · · · · · · ·
·
·
·

CHAPTER 3

Risk Factors for Developing Alzheimer's Disease

Lucky is he who has been able to
understand the cause of things.

Virgil

To treat or prevent a disease, it is helpful to identify its underlying causes. Since intensive research efforts first began in the late 1970s, there have been numerous theories about the underlying causes of AD. Environmental toxins, genetics, and viruses have all been suspected. Yet researchers have been frustrated in their efforts to understand the basic biological mechanisms that lead to AD, and no single cause for AD has been identified. There is a consensus among scientists that AD probably has many complex and related causes, similar to other major diseases like heart disease, cancer, and stroke. In this chapter I summarize key scientific findings about potential causes of AD and end with a look at the role of depression in the disease.

IDENTIFYING RISK FACTORS

Circumstances that put one at risk for developing diseases are referred to as "risk factors" or "susceptibility factors." A common risk factor for acquiring many diseases is exposure to environmental toxins. For example, inhaling tobacco smoke is well known to increase the risk of getting certain lung and heart diseases. Exposure to asbestos increases one's risk of developing cancer. High blood pressure, high cholesterol levels, and obesity significantly increase one's chances of developing heart disease. Identifying these risk factors in recent decades has led to major advances in prevention and treatment of heart disease.

Another common risk factor for developing disease involves genetics. Some defective genes or mutations can directly cause diseases while others increase susceptibility to certain diseases. For example, hereditary disorders such as cystic fibrosis and sickle-cell anemia are caused by transmission of specific genes from parent to child. Many such genetic disorders are easily identified through testing one's genetic makeup, or DNA. And although very few diseases pose a 100 percent risk of being transmitted from an affected parent to his or her children, a genetic susceptibility or vulnerability may be present among the vast majority of diseases. In other words, genetics may play a partial role in the development of most diseases but rarely seems to play an absolutely causative role. Most chronic diseases, including AD, are likely caused by a complex interaction of genetic and environmental risk factors.

For better or worse, we inherit a set of genes from both our mother and father that may protect or put us at risk for certain diseases. Advances in understanding human genetics may ultimately lead to ways of blocking the action of defective genes and promoting drugs that mimic genes with protective effects. In the meantime, the search continues for factors in the environment that put us at risk for certain diseases, including AD, so that we can modify our lifestyles and ward off these diseases. If reversible risk factors can be identified, we may discover clues about preventive measures and better treatments. We are just beginning to understand the risk factors for AD. Tantalizing research findings thus far highlight the importance of increased funding so that more intensive scientific investigations can take place.

DEFINITE RISK FACTORS

Although researchers have already identified several factors that definitely increase one's risk of developing AD, none of these can be altered, at least not yet. It is hoped that identifying other factors will help reduce the risk of developing AD. What has been known about the nature and progression of AD in the past has been based mainly on those severe cases that ordinarily come to the attention of physicians and others working in health-care centers. However, fuller understanding of the disease requires a closer look at the whole range of people affected by AD, who may live in the community by themselves or with the help of others. Over the past twenty years, large population studies conducted in the United States, Europe, and Japan have been useful in shedding light on risk factors for the disease. Table 3.1 lists currently known risk factors for AD; other possible factors will be addressed later.

Table 3.1: Definite Risk Factors for Alzheimer's Disease

- Advanced age
- Family history of AD/genetics
- Down's syndrome
- History of head trauma
- Low educational and occupational status

Advanced Age

As many studies have confirmed, there is an increased chance of getting AD as we grow older. In a widely respected community-based study of East Boston residents in the 1980s, researchers at Harvard Medical School found that 3 percent of those between the ages of sixty-five and seventy-four fit the criteria for probable AD; in the group between the ages seventy-five and eighty-four, nearly 19 percent showed signs of the disease; and in those aged eighty-five and older, 47 percent had symptoms of AD.[1] In effect, the risk of getting AD doubles about every five years after age sixty-five.

Based on reliable studies, it is now estimated that nearly five million Americans have the disease.[2] The World Health Organization estimates that 37 million worldwide have dementia.[3] Obviously, not all older people automatically get AD, so other risk factors play a role in the development of the disease.

Family History of AD/Genetics

As with other major diseases such as heart disease, cancer, and stroke, another risk factor for AD is having a first-degree blood relative with the disease, such as a parent, brother, or sister.[4] Although having a family history of the disease does not mean that one is destined to get it, hereditary factors may increase one's chances, that is, give one a genetic predisposition. It is well established that those who have a first-degree blood relative with the disease are one and a half to two times as likely to develop AD as those without a family history of the disease. Again, although risk is increased by a family history of AD, there is still no certainty of getting the disease.

On the other hand, in a very small number of cases, there is a definite genetic link in families whose members get the disease in middle age. This rare form of the disease is referred to as Familial AD, or the inherited "early-onset" form of AD. This form of the disease has been traced to genetic mutations on chromosomes 1, 14, and 21.[5] A mutation is passed from generation to generation in much the same way as it is in other genetic diseases such as cystic fibrosis and Huntington's disease, and these genetic mutations actually cause the disease. In Chapter 2, I noted that there is no foolproof diagnostic test for AD. These rare cases involving one of the three known genetic mutations linked to Familial AD, for which genetic testing does exist, are an exception to that rule. However, many ethical and legal issues are raised by the prospect of predictive testing for a disease that is not yet considered preventable.[6] Given the serious implications of genetic testing, counseling with a qualified professional both before and after testing is recommended.

People under sixty-five years of age represent a very small minority of the total number of people with AD, probably less than one percent. In most of these cases, there is no known genetic mutation. Several members of the same generation within a family may be affected by AD, or there may be only one member of the family with the disease. How the disease is transmitted in a family through yet unidentified mutations or why it may affect only one person in a family is not yet understood. Clearly, heredity alone does not explain the cause or causes of the disease. Although there is growing evidence that heredity plays a stronger role in the development of AD than was previously suspected, AD is not considered a true genetic disorder except in the rare familial form of the disease described above. Here the distinction between genetic "susceptibility" and "certainty" is key.

The more common variety of AD is the "late-onset" form, which occurs among people aged sixty-five and older and has been linked to one gene thus far. In 1993, researchers at Duke University Medical Center discovered that the presence of a specific gene that controls the production of a protein is a major risk factor for AD.[7] This gene is found on chromosome 19. The protein, known as apolipoprotein, or ApoE, is involved in transporting cholesterol in the blood. ApoE comes in three types, and one of these types is inherited from each biological parent. People born with a type of the gene known as ApoE4 run a higher risk of getting AD than those born with other types of the gene, known as ApoE2 and ApoE3. But clearly the gene for ApoE4 does not convey the disease to every person who inherits it. Likewise, it is also well known that those without the gene may also develop AD.

Although ApoE4 is an important risk factor for AD, it accounts for only a portion of people with the disease.[8] Therefore, other genetic and environmental risk factors must be at work. Other susceptibility genes have been reported in relation to AD but only the ApoE4 gene has been confirmed as a susceptibility factor thus far. In recent years, researchers have been looking for another susceptibility gene on chromosome 10.[9] Although another specific gene has not yet been pinpointed, it is highly likely that more than one gene makes older people more susceptible to developing AD. Quite clearly, genetics plays an important part in the development of AD.

Measuring susceptibility to AD might be of interest to people with a family history of the disease, and those most at risk might opt for trying preventive measures. But although a blood test is available for determining one's type of ApoE, this information cannot accurately measure risk or susceptibility and so has very limited value. The Alzheimer's Association, as well as several medical societies, has not yet recommended any test as accurately predicting or diagnosing the common late-onset form of AD.[10] For now, the ApoE blood test and other means to ascertain a diagnosis are considered tools for researchers, not valid diagnostic tests.

Technological advances may eventually make it possible to determine one's risk of getting AD and a host of other diseases with great accuracy. However, any truly predictive biological test is bound to pose dilemmas for those who are susceptible, since there is currently no effective way to prevent AD. Would it be helpful to know that AD lies in one's future, perhaps many decades away? Would foreknowledge of the disease affect choices about marriage, children, and career? Would it be possible to obtain long-term-care insurance if there were a strong probability that care would be needed in the future? Such questions already face many families with known hereditary disorders. Nevertheless, advances in predictive testing raise profound questions, and scientific progress could soon outpace society's ability to arrive at satisfactory answers.

Genetic studies currently being conducted at research centers throughout the world may ultimately identify additional genes that play a part in the development of AD. The mammoth Human Genome Project sponsored by the U.S. government successfully cataloged the entire complement of DNA in human genes. Related projects may yield further clues about the genetic origins of AD. Pinpointing genes linked to AD could theoretically target the development of gene-based or drug treatments. In theory, people at high risk could be identified before symptoms of AD unfold in an effort to delay or prevent its onset. Today, progress toward such ambitious goals is just beginning and expectations are high for breakthroughs in the future.

Down's Syndrome

Another genetic risk factor concerns people with Down's syndrome, a form of mental retardation linked to chromosome 21. When their brains are examined under a microscope at an autopsy, virtually all middle-aged people with Down's syndrome exhibit changes in brain tissue consistent with AD.[11] For reasons that are unknown, however, not all people with Down's syndrome manifest the classic symptoms of AD during their lifetimes, although prevalence of the disease increases significantly after age forty.[12] In other words, the expression of AD symptoms among people with Down's syndrome is substantially less than would be expected, given the high prevalence of AD confirmed at autopsy. The reasons for this discrepancy are not yet fully understood.

History of Head Trauma

One factor that presents a real risk for developing AD is a history of head trauma. It is well known that professional boxers who suffer repeated blows to the head are at high risk of impairments to their memory, language, and other brain functions. Several studies have also shown that suffering a severe blow to the head resulting in loss of consciousness increases the risk of developing AD later in life.[13] It has also been shown that even a minor head injury occurring early in life may have a lasting effect that predisposes one to AD late in life.[14] Just how large a risk this injury poses has not yet been clearly defined but a history of head trauma presents a definite risk for developing AD.

Low Educational and Occupational Status

A major area of study concerns the relation between the risk of AD and one's level of education and occupation. There is now convincing evidence that people with low educational and occupational attainment are at greater risk of developing AD than the general population.[15] Conversely, those with high educational and occupational attainment may be at lower risk for developing AD.

Several explanations have been put forth about how education and occupation play a role in the development of AD. First, higher-educated people perform better on tests of intellectual ability than others and are not as easily identified as having symptoms of AD. Second, higher levels of education may somehow increase the number of connections among brain cells, reducing the manifestations of the disease in susceptible individuals. Since education and occupation are linked to socioeconomic status, other lifestyle factors such as diet and smoking must certainly be considered. Furthermore, since formal education takes place primarily early in life, the role of childhood development cannot be overlooked in determining the risk for disease later in life. Whether low levels of education or occupation are true risk factors or whether they represent markers for other disease-related factors will not be known until further research is done.

Studies concerning education and occupation suggest that people who tax their brains throughout their lives may reduce their risk of developing AD. Yet the fact that people with keen intellects may develop AD demonstrates that they are not immune to the disease. Prime examples include renowned artists Norman Rockwell and Willem de Kooning and the acclaimed author and philosopher Dame Iris Murdoch. It remains to be seen whether high educational and occupational attainment may truly protect against AD to some degree, and conversely, whether low educational and occupational attainment may increase the risk of developing the disease.

In summary, there are many factors definitely associated with an increased risk of developing AD, such as advanced age, family history, genetics, head trauma, and low educational and occupational attainment. Researchers continue to look for other risk factors that might be modified so we can decrease or eliminate the risk of developing AD.

POSSIBLE RISK FACTORS

Possible risk factors (see Table 3.2) are those suspected of being somehow linked to AD but not yet proven to have a consistent association with the disease. Additional research is needed to clarify their role, since studies about these possible factors have not been thoroughly carried out. There is considerable speculation over how much or how little these factors influence the development of AD. Nevertheless, identifying just one factor that could be modified to reduce the risk of developing AD would have enormous implications. For example, if it were known for certain that a particular food or chemical increases the risk of developing the disease, such things could be avoided and the number of people with AD could be substantially reduced.

Table 3.2: Possible Risk Factors for Alzheimer's Disease

» Female gender
» Small strokes or cerebrovascular disease
» Parkinson's disease
» Race and ethnicity
» Environmental toxins
» Diet
» Lack of exercise
» High cholesterol
» Stress
» Depression before onset of AD

Female Gender

One possible risk factor for developing AD is inborn: being female. It is a fact that the vast majority of people with AD are women. Of course, women tend to live longer than men do, and the disease is strongly related to advanced age. However, some studies have shown that even when longevity is taken into account, women still have a greater chance than men of developing AD.[16] There is speculation among researchers regarding this disparity. One theory is that decreasing levels of estrogen as women age may be somehow related to an increased susceptibility to AD. But clearly this natural part of the aging process is probably not the sole reason for women possibly being at greater risk of developing AD than men.

Small Strokes or Cerebrovascular Disease

Another possible risk factor concerns tiny strokes or infarcts in the brain. Several studies, which looked at brain scans or at brain tissue after death, suggest a small number of brain infarcts can make it more likely for people to express the symptoms of AD. For example, in a large study of American Catholic nuns, those who had suffered tiny strokes had a much higher risk of developing symptoms of AD during their lifetime than those who had not experienced this type of brain damage.[17] This finding was remarkable in that strokes associated with the small blood vessels in the brain are potentially treatable and preventable. Additional findings from this study and similar ones should yield more definitive results in the near future about the role that small strokes play in the development of AD. In the meantime, steps to prevent strokes should be taken, such as keeping blood pressure under control and avoiding tobacco smoke; a physician should be consulted about additional steps.

Parkinson's Disease

Another medical condition that appears to pose a risk for developing AD is Parkinson's disease, a neurological disorder that impairs the movement of hands, arms, and legs. Between 20 and 30 percent of people with Parkinson's disease develop symptoms of AD, typically in the late stages of the disease.[18] Likewise, most people in the late stages of AD develop some symptoms of Parkinson's disease. The relationship between these two brain diseases is not yet fully understood.

Race and Ethnicity

Race and ethnicity have also been identified as possible risk factors for developing AD. One study showed that African Americans had five times the rate of dementia compared to European

Americans.[19] A large population study conducted in New York in the 1990s revealed that African Americans and Hispanics of Caribbean origin were at a much greater risk for AD than were members of other racial groups.[20] In this study, African Americans were four times more likely than European Americans to develop AD by age ninety, an increase that was shown to be unrelated to differences in education levels. It has been suggested that other genetic and environmental factors may determine the disproportionate rate of AD among these racial and ethnic groups. This theory is further supported by several recent studies. One large study showed higher rates of dementia among Japanese men who emigrated to Hawaii as compared to those who remained in Japan.[21] Additional large-scale studies will clarify the role of race and ethnicity as risk factors for AD and have implications for the general population.

Environmental Toxins

There are several theories about environmental triggers for AD, but no one trigger has been clearly identified as a true causative agent. Since ingestion of toxic metals such as lead can cause brain damage, there has been a vigorous search for something in the environment or something that we eat or breathe that may be a culprit. For many years the relationship between aluminum and AD was studied intensively, but is no longer a major consideration due to weak evidence that aluminum is a risk factor.[22] Other trace metals such as mercury found in dental fillings, zinc, and iron have shown no significant association with increased risk for AD.[23] Nevertheless, there may still be many unidentified chemicals or other toxic substances in the environment that play a role in the development of AD.

A U.S. study showed an increased risk of AD among people exposed to organic solvents such as benzene and toluene.[24] A Canadian study showed an increased risk for AD in those whose jobs expose them to glues, pesticides, and fertilizers.[25] A couple of small studies have suggested that exposure to electromagnetic fields may put people at risk for AD.[26] Although provocative, the results of such studies are not really conclusive and should be considered preliminary. Caution should always be exercised in interpreting the findings of studies that specify causes or risks for AD. Recent studies have suggested that cigarette smoking may increase the risk of developing AD. A large study by a Dutch team of researchers strongly suggests that cigarette smoking is an environmental culprit in the development of AD.[27] The study involved more than 6,800 men and women aged fifty-five and older, and those who smoked cigarettes were found to be more than twice as likely to develop AD than were those who didn't smoke. This study needs to be replicated before firm conclusions can be drawn about the exact role of smoking in increasing the risk for AD. Data pooled from four large European studies also showed that smoking contributes to memory loss in older people.[28] The role of smoking in causing or contributing to the development of a long list of diseases, such as lung cancer and heart disease, has already been well documented, and perhaps AD may one day be added to this list. It should be noted, however, that controversy exists on this point. Some studies have suggested that cigarette smoking may actually protect against the development of AD.[29] The many health risks of smoking certainly outweigh any potential benefits, but it is theorized that the protective benefit of smoking seen in these studies may be due to nicotine's possible role in enhancing memory. Consequently, the value of nicotine in treating AD has received attention by researchers.[30]

Diet

While the role of diet has received much attention in relation to other diseases, the potential role of diet in the development of AD has just recently received scientific investigation. Vitamin deficiency is known to cause a rare form of dementia, but unlike the dementia associated with AD, this condition can be treated and reversed. It has also been suggested that high intake of calories and fatty foods increase one's risk for developing AD.[31] In addition, several teams of researchers have found that high blood levels of the amino acid homocysteine and low blood levels of folic acid and other B vitamins are associated with increased susceptibility for AD.[32] Such possible risk factors are intriguing and deserve further investigation since they may be modified by diet and dietary supplements.

Lack of Exercise

Another possible and treatable risk factor for AD is lack of exercise. One team of researchers reported that those with AD exercised less between the ages of twenty and fifty-nine than those who did not develop AD late in life, and a Canadian study showed that regular physical activity was associated with a reduced risk of Alzheimer's disease.[33] It is logical to assume that our lifestyle habits, such as diet and exercise, play a role in health conditions that we develop in our later years. AD may be no exception to this general rule. Although exercise is known to be beneficial for the heart and lungs, the effects on the brain have not yet been proven. Preliminary findings offer hope that physical exercise is a fairly simple means of delaying or slowing down the onset of AD.

High Cholesterol

Related to the issues of diet and exercise are recent research findings that high cholesterol levels in the blood may also be a risk factor for AD.[34] High cholesterol is commonly known as a risk factor for cardiovascular disease and may also prove to be a treatable risk factor for AD. Proper diet, medications, physical exercise, and other lifestyle changes can lower cholesterol levels. There is now a great deal of research examining possible links between heart disease, stroke, and AD in order to find ways of preventing and treating these major diseases.

Stress

Psychological stress caused by major life events, such as the death of a loved one or divorce, is another possible risk factor, although there is controversy about the relationship between stress and AD. One large European study showed no association.[35] In some cases, where it appears that an individual developed AD right after a major life change, like the death of a spouse or retirement, close examination usually reveals that the person was developing the disease earlier but symptoms were not recognized or taken seriously. The role of stress in the development of AD is also being investigated among military veterans suffering from a combat-related condition known as "post-traumatic stress disorder." Some researchers report abnormal brain chemistry and impaired brain functions among such veterans.[36] While these findings are intriguing, the possible role of stress in the development of AD in the general population is not yet known.

Depression Before Onset of AD

Another possible risk factor for AD is an affected person's history of depression before the onset of AD. There is evidence that some people with AD exhibit depressive symptoms before they show the classic symptoms of the disease, such as loss of recent memory.[37] These people may make vague complaints about lack of energy, loss of interest, or "not feeling right." Their close relatives and friends may notice subtle changes in their personality or behavior. However, formal testing typically reveals no significant abnormalities in their memory and thinking abilities. Over a period of several years, however, their depression may persist in spite of treatment with antidepressant medication and/or counseling. Eventually, they manifest the more classic symptoms of AD. Whether or not depression represents a true risk factor or heralds the onset of AD remains unclear. Since depression is fairly common among older adults and is often confused with the early stages of AD, it is a topic that warrants further discussion.

EXPLORING THE ROLE OF DEPRESSION

According to the National Institutes of Health, depressive symptoms occur in about 15 percent of people aged sixty-five and older, and major depression affects just under 3 percent of older Americans.[38] Symptoms of depression may include irritability, crying spells, apathy, difficulty concentrating or remembering, sleep disturbance, fatigue, problems with eating (weight gain or loss), diminished interest in pleasurable activities including sex, and feelings of worthlessness and hopelessness. Since AD and depression share some symptoms, people with AD are sometimes misdiagnosed at first. Depression can also coexist with AD, with estimates suggesting that from 11 to 50 percent of people with AD also exhibit signs of depression.[39] Confusion arises because some people who are depressed show symptoms that may mimic the early stages of AD, and some people in the early stages of the disease may also be depressed over their failing abilities. In either case, physicians often prescribe antidepressant medications. Those whose root problem is actually depression will probably experience an improvement in their mood as well as in their memory and thinking, while those whose root problem is AD and who are not depressed will probably not experience any improvement in their memory and thinking.

There are at least two interrelated causes of depression: psychological disturbance and biological changes. Depression is a normal psychological reaction to loss. For people with AD, loss of intellectual abilities occurs gradually. Those with a high level of awareness about their disease may be understandably depressed about these losses. A growing dependency on others because of limitations imposed by AD may diminish their self-esteem. They may worry about being abandoned, even by their devoted spouse. They may feel guilty about the perceived burden that the disease places on others. They may feel alienated and sense that people are treating them differently. Whether or not these thoughts and feelings seem rational, they should not be taken lightly. Affected people's subjective experience of the disease may be quite real and painful.

In addition to a psychological reaction to the personal losses associated with AD, depression may also be caused by chemical changes in the brain. It is well known that people with AD have reduced levels of many brain chemicals, including serotonin.[40] It is also known that a reduced level of serotonin is associated with major depression. Regardless of the underlying cause, every effort should be made to alleviate symptoms of depression. The decision to obtain an evaluation and treatment for depression should not be left solely to the person with AD. Rather, others close to the affected person often must take the initiative so that a physician may properly evaluate and treat the problem.

Numerous antidepressant medications are now available that are relatively safe and effective in relieving symptoms of depression. Although psychiatrists have traditionally been consulted to prescribe and monitor these medications, primary care physicians have become increasingly familiar with these medications in recent years. They may feel comfortable treating their depressed patients with a class of drugs known as Selective Serotonin Reuptake Inhibitors, or SSRIs, that are designed to increase the level of serotonin in the brain. SSRIs have fewer side effects than the traditional antidepressants known as tricyclics. SSRIs include brand names like Zoloft, Paxil, Prozac, Luvox, and, more recently, Celexa. In 1998, a consensus panel of American experts recommended sertraline (Zoloft) and paroxetine (Paxil) as first-line choices of treatment for depression among older people who also have AD or a related dementia.[41] Because responses to drugs vary from person to person, different types of drugs and different dosages may have to be tried before improvement is seen. A physician must count on the cooperation of the person being treated as well as close observers to monitor responses to treatment. Again, although an affected person's mood is expected to lift with treatment of depression, memory impairment and other difficulties caused by AD usually are not expected to improve.

Controversy exists over the value of individual or group therapy for people with AD who are also depressed. Since the disease affects the capacity to create and retain new memories, the benefits derived from talk therapy may be nonexistent or limited. Carrying over ideas and insights from one therapy session to the next can obviously be challenging for someone whose memory is impaired. Thus far there is no convincing evidence that persons with coexistent AD and depression benefit from counseling. Despite the lack of studies proving the benefits of group and individual counseling, such help may be beneficial in some cases. Medicare, the federal health insurance system in the United States for most older adults and younger disabled adults, covers the cost of counseling for people with AD by certified mental health professionals. If talk therapy is going to be useful for an individual with AD, it is more likely to help in the early stages of the disease than in later stages.

The elderly population is growing rapidly and living longer than ever before. As a result, the number of people with AD is projected to increase dramatically in coming decades—unless major scientific advances help control this increase. Although aging is not a reversible risk factor despite what "anti-aging" advocates claim, other factors may be identified in the future that can enable us to modify our lifestyle and lower the risk of developing the disease. Attempts to associate AD with environmental toxins, viruses, personality types, health habits, or lifestyles have met with some success thus far. Just as it took a long time to identify certain lifestyle habits that influence the personal risk of heart disease, the same is likely to happen with AD. Most researchers now believe that AD is similar to other common diseases in that it is caused by interrelated factors, both genetic and environmental.

It is evident that many factors intersect and set in motion a complex cascade of events inside the brain before symptoms of AD actually appear. Researchers are slowly gaining insights into the underlying biology of the disease and potentially reversible, treatable risk factors. We know that many chemical systems in the brain are affected in different ways in AD, so no single cure or "magic bullet" is likely to be found. In the next chapter, I will discuss current and future trends in treating and preventing the disease.

. . . .

.

.

.

CHAPTER 4

Progress in
Treatment and
Prevention of
Alzheimer's Disease

*Every complex problem has a
solution that is simple, neat, and
wrong.*

H. L. Mencken

In this chapter I will review current options for treating AD as
well as some options that may become available in the future
for treating, slowing down, and preventing the disease.
Although there is still little that can be done to dramatically
improve symptoms or slow down the progression of AD, some
potentially useful drug treatments have recently become available
or are on the horizon. These include antidementia drugs that are
in testing phases at research centers, mainly in North America,
Europe, and Japan. And although claims that certain herbs and
dietary supplements may enhance memory have not yet been sub-
stantiated, in spite of their growing popularity, some alternative
medicines may also prove beneficial.

It seems that the media report on a new study about AD
almost every month. However, most of these studies have no

immediate applicability to people with the disease. For example, despite important new research on the brain's ability to regenerate cells and a potential vaccine for AD, it remains to be seen if these findings yield any real benefits for people with the disease. Likewise, advances in gene therapy and cell transplantation for diseases affecting the brain have no relevance for people with AD in the near future. Therefore, we should be careful about reading too much into these preliminary reports. However, real progress in the treatment of AD is beginning to be made.

Currently there are no antidementia drugs that can benefit everyone with AD. Some of these drugs have received approval from the United States government or are being considered for approval by the Food and Drug Administration (FDA). These drugs are modestly beneficial for less than half the people in the early and middle stages of AD. Although their benefits are usually short-lived, there is some evidence that they may also have longer-lasting effects. Because there is no way to predict who may benefit from these drugs, each individual with AD who can afford it should probably take a course of one of these drugs on a trial basis to determine its effectiveness. As with all other drugs, they should be taken under the supervision of a competent and experienced physician who can help you in assessing the safety and effectiveness of the treatment.

Most drugs tested so far for AD are attempts to replace chemicals that are deficient in the brains of people with AD. This approach follows the model used in treating Parkinson's disease, another common brain disorder among older people that results in slowed movements, rigidity, and tremors. Deficiency of a chemical called dopamine is chiefly responsible for the symptoms of Parkinson's. There are several prescription drugs available that attempt to compensate for this deficiency, and as a result, people with Parkinson's disease often find relief, sometimes even dramatic improvement, of their symptoms. The problem with a single-drug approach to treating AD is that there is a whole host of deficiencies in the brains of people with the disease. No single drug has been developed that is capable of replenishing all these chemicals.

CURRENT TREATMENTS

So far, after rigorous testing over a period of many years, only four drug treatments for AD have been approved by the FDA. These antidementia drugs are available only through a written prescription. Other drugs are in various phases of testing in the United States and elsewhere, and their entry into the marketplace is expected in the next few years. Table 4.1 lists the four drugs and their respective recommended dosage.

Table 4.1: Treatments for Alzheimer's Disease Approved by the FDA*

Drug Name / Brand Name	Manufacturer	Current Status	Manufacturer's Recommended Dosage
Tacrine/ Cognex	Parke-Davis	Approved in 1994; no longer actively marketed	10mg four times/day (40mg/day); increase by 40mg/day every day to 40mg four times a day (160mg/day)
Donepezil/ Aricep	Eisai, Inc.	Approved in 1996	5mg once a day; increase after four to six weeks to 10mg once a day
Rivastigmine/ Exelon	Novartis Pharmaceuticals	Approved in 2000	1.5mg twice a day (3mg/day); increase by 3mg/day every two weeks to 6mg twice a day (12mg/day)
Galantamine/ Reminyl	Janssen Pharmaceutical Products	Approved in 2001	4mg twice daily (8mg/day); increase by 8mg/day after four weeks to 8mg twice a day (16mg/day)

* Information current as of February 2003.

Cholinesterase Inhibitors

All of the drugs currently approved for the treatment of AD in the United States belong to a class known as cholinesterase inhibitors. These prescription drugs work basically by delaying or inhibiting the breakdown of a key brain chemical called acetylcholine. This class of drugs essentially aims to artificially mimic a process that occurs naturally. Evidence to date indicates that all of these drugs have modest but meaningful effects on about half of those in the early and middle stages of AD.[1] Benefits include slight improvement for a period of many months in memory, language skills, and ability to handle tasks like personal grooming. There is evidence that these drugs may help to slow one's expected rate of decline. In effect, they may be equivalent to "turning back the clock" in the disease process by six months, or even longer in some cases.[2] Thus, these drugs potentially prolong one's independence for a longer period of time than expected without their use. Again, not everyone responds favorably to these drugs, so expectations should be tempered.

Benefits reported for these drugs tend to occur at higher doses that also increase the likelihood of known side effects such as diarrhea, vomiting, and nausea. In light of the potential for such adverse gastrointestinal effects, interaction with nonsteroidal anti-inflammatory drugs (NSAIDs) such as Advil and Motrin is cautioned since this class of prescription and over-the-counter drugs can cause similar problems. (See the section on anti-inflammatory drugs, later in this chapter, for more information on NSAIDS.) As with any type of drug, careful monitoring is required with all of the cholinesterase inhibitors. Due to their potential for slowing the progression of AD, these drugs are being tested to see if they might delay the onset of the disease among people with mild cognitive impairment (MCI).

There is no evidence to support the idea that combining these drugs would be any more beneficial than taking one alone. Moreover, a combination of these drugs is bound to increase the chance of unwanted side effects. Perhaps a new class of drugs will be better taken in combination with the current class of drugs. Although a study directly comparing the current class of antidementia drugs might be useful in determining which one is most beneficial over a longer time, no such study has yet been completed. The only way to determine which drug is better for a particular person is simply trial and error. Although the drugs operate in similar ways on the brain, they have different chemical properties, side effects, and safety profiles. Individuals with AD often respond differently to the drugs, so it is important to keep an open mind during the trial-and-error process. There is some evidence that if one drug is not effective or is not well tolerated, switching to another one might be beneficial.[3]

What are the practical benefits of the antidementia drugs now available? Again, about half the people in the early and middle stages of AD who take them respond favorably, at least for a while, either in terms of improvement or stability. Improvements in memory, thinking, and concentration are the most frequently reported positive changes. Family members report that the affected person often seems "sharper" or more attentive during drug treatment. The person's ability to recall recent events and to complete personal care and household tasks may also improve. Problems such as repeating questions, misplacing objects, or becoming confused in new surroundings may be eased, and mood and behavior may also be improved. Although the changes are seldom dramatic, the families of those with AD are usually grateful. Because it is tempting to look for improvement even where none exists, the true effectiveness of a particular drug should be medically evaluated after it has been tried for a few months.

One practical consideration is the cost of these drugs. All of them cost about four to five dollars a day, an expense that may be difficult for many people, especially if they need other drugs for other health problems. The health insurance plan of the person with AD may offer full or partial coverage of these medications. Currently, Medicare does not cover these or any other medications except for inpatient use, but the combined federal and state medical assistance program for poor people, known as Medicaid, does cover them. The state agency that administers this program locally is usually the department of human services. Also, more than fifteen states in the United States have set up programs to help pay for the cost of drugs among near-poor elderly and disabled people. Check with your state's department of health to find out if such a program is available. For those who do not qualify for the above programs and cannot afford the drugs, the companies who make them have set up assistance programs so that the drugs may be received free through one's physician. You should be able to obtain an application form and information about each company's eligibility criteria from your physician. For a free copy of the current issue of the "Directory of Prescription Drug Patient Assistance Programs," write to: PhRMA (Pharmaceutical Research and Manufacturers of America), 1100 Fifteenth Street NW, Washington, DC, 20005. This directory is also available on the Internet (see Internet Resources under "Other Websites of Interest").

PROGRESS IN TREATMENT AND PREVENTION

There may be as many as two dozen drugs for Alzheimer's disease in various phases of testing at research centers throughout the world. It may take several years before the value of these experimental drugs is fully understood. All of them are attempts to improve upon the performance of the pioneering antidementia drugs already approved by the FDA. In the coming years, we should see a number of additional antidementia drugs offering more meaningful and longer-lasting benefits to people with AD.

Table 4.2: Approaches to Treating, Slowing, or Preventing Alzheimer's Disease

Cholinesterase inhibitors

 ▸ Anti-inflammatory drugs
 ▸ Statin drugs
 ▸ Estrogen-replacement therapy

Antioxidants

 ▸ Other complementary and alternative medicine
 ▸ The "use-it-or-lose-it" approach
 ▸ A vaccine?

Table 4.2 above lists several approaches to treat, delay, or prevent the onset of Alzheimer's disease that are in various phases of study.[4] Since preventing the disease is obviously far more desirable than simply treating its symptoms, it is likely that prevention will be a major focus of research in the future.

Anti-Inflammatory Drugs

Researchers know that inflammation in the brain contributes to AD, so it is logical to consider the role of anti-inflammatory drugs in preventing or treating the disease. There is preliminary evidence suggesting that regular use of nonsteroidal anti-inflammatory drugs (NSAIDs), including the prescription drugs (Indocin, Celebrex, and Vioxx), and over-the-counter drugs such as ibuprofen (Motrin, Advil) and naproxen sodium (Aleve), may protect against AD. Several studies have shown that people who take NSAIDs for treating arthritis are less likely to develop AD than people who do not.[5] Consequently, researchers are now examining the potential role of NSAIDs in delaying the onset of the disease among older people with mild cognitive impairment. The use of NSAIDs in treating people already with AD is not fully known but a large study involving two different NSAIDs recently proved disappointing.[6] Also, in light of their potential side effects, NSAIDs are not now recommended for treating or preventing AD.

Statin Drugs

Recent studies have shown that people who take statins, a class of drugs that lowers cholesterol, have a significantly reduced risk of AD compared with those who take other cholesterol-lowering agents or no such drug at all.[7] Cholesterol-lowering drugs are known to help ward off and treat coronary artery disease and stroke. Their potential use in relation to AD lends credence to a theory regarding links between cardiovascular disease and AD. How statin drugs actually work to reduce the risk of AD is not known. Statins now marketed in the United States include lovastatin, atorvastatin, fluvastatin, pravastatin and many others. There is considerable excitement about large clinical trials now in progress that will determine if statins are indeed useful in cutting the risk of AD and treating those in the early and middle stages of the disease.

Estrogen-Replacement Therapy

Despite encouraging findings from preliminary studies, clinical trials show that estrogen-replacement therapy does not appear to prevent AD or slow its progression among women following menopause.[8] Further tests involving the role of estrogen in treating or preventing AD are in progress, and whether estrogen might be beneficial for some women remains to be seen. However, estrogen use in the general population is likely to diminish in light of widely publicized findings from an American study showing serious adverse effects among some women.[9]

Antioxidants

Research suggests that the death of brain cells occurring in people with AD partially results from the increased production of "free radicals," oxygen molecules that cause damage throughout the body.[10] There has been a great deal of speculation about the potential benefits of antioxidants in slowing down and preventing this damage. Many studies are beginning to examine this approach to preventing and treating AD. Preliminary studies look promising.

In a major study that tested high doses of a common antioxidant, vitamin E, among people in the middle to late stages of AD, those who took supplemental vitamin E at about seventy times the recommended daily dosage experienced some beneficial effects.[11] In this study, a dosage of 2,000 international units of vitamin E daily slowed down the expected rate of decline compared to those in a control group, who received a placebo. Although the results of the study were not conclusive, many physicians now recommend that those with AD take high doses of vitamin E, since it is potentially beneficial, relatively safe, and inexpensive. The only caveat is that a high dose of vitamin E is potentially harmful if combined with blood-thinning drugs.

Two large studies have shown that older people who regularly got ample amounts of vitamin E or C *through food but not supplements*, significantly lowered their risk of developing AD.[12] Current studies of antioxidants including supplemental folate, selenium, vitamin B6, and vitamin B12 are examining if the rate of decline can be slowed among people with AD. These nutrients are naturally found in green, leafy vegetables but are also available as nutritional supplements in over-the-counter products. Folic acid and B vitamins are considered good products for further study since they are both safe and inexpensive.

Other antioxidants have also shown some promise. For example, gingko biloba extract, taken from the leaves of the gingko tree, was reportedly slightly effective in treating people with AD and other dementias.[13] Due to major flaws in the study, however, its findings were questionable. A formal review of several studies showed a small but significant effect of treatment with 120 to 240 mg of gingko biloba daily.[14] At present, a large clinical trial of gingko biloba, funded by the National Center for Complementary and Alternative Medicine, is taking place at numerous sites throughout the United States that will clarify the role of gingko in treating AD. Although Germany has approved gingko extracts (240 mg a day) to treat AD, and gingko biloba has been used for 5,000 years in traditional Chinese medicine for various purposes, there is not yet consensus among North American physicians about its value in treating AD.

With respect to memory, many preliminary studies involving animals have shown the benefits of certain foods, such as spinach, blueberries, and strawberries, that are loaded with antioxidants. Whether such findings apply to humans still remains to be seen. Although nutrition alone is clearly not a sufficient treatment for AD, keeping a healthy diet is always a good idea.

Other Complementary and Alternative Medicine

Because there are no major medical treatments for AD and the pace of research is slow, many people seek help outside the scientific mainstream. More and more people have become disillusioned about the limits of modern medicine in treating a variety of conditions and illnesses. Ancient practices such as acupuncture, acupressure, massage, aromatherapy, and herbal medicine have seen a resurgence. Billions of dollars are spent annually in the United States on alternative therapies. Many practitioners of complementary and alternative medicine claim to offer help and healing to those with medical conditions unresponsive to conventional treatments. Perhaps modern science will some day prove that some of these unorthodox therapies actually work. The interest in alternative medicine is bound to grow with the aging of the baby boom generation. The National Center for Complementary and Alternative Medicine, under the auspices of the National Institutes of Health, is charged with investigating these old and new forms of treatment (call [888] 644-6226 or see Internet Resources for further information).

The makers of such products have proposed many dietary supplements, herbal remedies, and other natural agents for improving memory or increasing blood flow to the brain. Hormones such as DHEA and herbal medicines such as garlic, ginseng, kava, and green tea have been touted as memory enhancers or as natural means of improving concentration. These products can be sold in the United States without meeting the stringent guidelines the FDA sets for drugs, as long as the sellers do not claim to treat, cure, or prevent disease. Their popularity and huge sales indicate a widespread belief that there must be some advantages to these forms of alternative medicine. However, there have been no controlled studies thus far to either prove or disprove claims of effectiveness for any of these products, and consumers may not have reliable information about their safety, effectiveness, or potency.

There have been claims that a natural product known as huperzine, an extract derived from a Chinese club-moss plant that is a traditional Chinese herbal remedy for fever, enhances memory and concentration. Huperzine has similar chemical properties to the current class of antidementia drugs (cholinesterase inhibitors) approved in the United States, and these claims seem to have some scientific basis, as evidenced in preliminary studies on rats and humans.[15] Because huperzine is considered a dietary supplement and therefore is not within the realm of FDA regulation, it is available over the counter in nutrition stores throughout the United States. However, it probably deserves the kind of monitoring normally reserved for prescription drugs, according to some experts.[16] Fortunately, a government-sponsored study of huperzine will soon be taking place in the United States to determine its safety and effectiveness in treating AD.

Although the desire to try out the vast array of available alternative treatments is understandable, it is also important to retain a healthy skepticism about unproven pills, procedures, and practices. There are many well-meaning people who believe that they have stumbled on a breakthrough without the benefit of rigorous methods to test their claims. Likewise, there are unscrupulous opportunists eager to prey on the vulnerability of people who are desperate for anything of potential value. If you are interested in pursuing alternative therapies, it is recommended you do so with a buyer-beware mentality. In pinning your hopes on a quick fix for AD, you run the risk of both disappointment and exploitation.

The "Use-It-or-Lose-It" Approach

Questions often arise about the value of mental exercises in preventing brain diseases or in increasing "brain power." This use-it-or-lose-it theory is gaining increased attention in scientific circles. Brain researchers are now finding that nerve cells in mammals' brains continue to generate long after maturation, suggesting that similar cell generation is probable in humans. Moreover, scientists are beginning to explore the effects of impoverished versus enriched environments on the brain. Through experiments with rodents, researchers in recent years have demonstrated that lack of mental stimulation reduces the number of brain cells, whereas increased stimulation promotes the growth of new brain cells.[17] Recent human studies have shown that mental stimulation later in life may play a key role in delaying or preventing AD.[18] Many intellectual exercises, such as playing cards or chess, reading a book, taking a class, or learning a new hobby, are both interesting and pleasurable. Personal satisfaction alone makes these activities appealing, and whether they ward off AD to some extent or not, there is no harm in using them to keep mentally active.

There is no clear evidence so far, though, that training or exercising brain functions such as memory has any benefits for people with AD. Once brain cells have been damaged or destroyed by the disease, they cannot be restored through strenuous effort. Nor do mental exercises appear to keep healthy brain cells functioning for a longer time. Memory exercises can actually be counterproductive among people with AD in certain situations, since pressure to remember things may trigger frustration and lower an affected person's self-esteem. However, different types of stimulation have been shown to affect the mood and behavior of people with AD. For example, a loud and overstimulating environment can be agitating, while soothing music is known to have a calming effect on people with the disease. Ideas concerning suitable mental and physical activities for people in the early stages of AD are addressed in Chapter 10.

A Vaccine?

Clearly, a vaccine to treat or prevent AD would represent a quantum leap forward in medicine. An experimental vaccine for AD, used successfully in laboratory mice, gained much public attention in 1999, but a human trial was halted in 2001 due to serious adverse effects. Whether a reformulated vaccine will be attempted again remains to be seen but several research firms are exploring this approach.

Although the chance of dramatic progress being made in the treatment or prevention of AD cannot be discounted, smaller or gradual advances are more likely. Hope lies in all the research being conducted by scientists throughout the world, especially in the United States, the leader in AD research. The speed at which treatment and prevention efforts are developed is generally related to the level of funding for research. Private funding of AD research has risen significantly in recent years. Yet sadly, federal funding of AD research in the United States remains relatively low, despite the enormous economic and human costs of the problem. As a result, progress is relatively slow. Advocates of an accelerated research initiative must push this agenda forward with public officials while continuing to raise funds for privately backed research efforts. Another way to get involved directly in such efforts is to participate as a volunteer in research programs.

PARTICIPATING IN CLINICAL DRUG TRIALS AND OTHER STUDIES

Any new drug intended to treat people ultimately has to be tested on people in clinical trials, which determine if it is safe and effective, at what doses it works best, and what side effects it has. Standards for effectiveness and safety differ in each country. The FDA in the United States is perhaps the most stringent regulatory agency of any government in the world, in an effort to ensure that all drugs meet the highest standards for safety and effectiveness through different phases of clinical testing.

Someone with AD may want to consider enrolling in one of the many drug trials being conducted at different places in the United States, or in other types of research studies. An obvious and legitimate reason for participating is self-interest. Studies offering the potential of direct, personal benefits are most appealing. Participation in research may also provide opportunities to become better educated about AD, to discuss ways of coping, and to feel supported by the professionals conducting the studies. Such benefits may be of interest to the person with AD and loved ones.

The research that is often of most interest to people with AD and their families concerns experimental drugs. If the antidementia treatments you have encountered prove disappointing, then you may wish to enroll in a study of a newer, experimental drug. This may offer you reassurance that everything possible is being tried. The early stage of the disease is the proper time to consider this option, since people in later stages are typically excluded from participation for a variety of medical, legal, and ethical reasons.

Clinical trials of new drugs are conducted in several phases over a period of many years, usually under the auspices of a pharmaceutical company. Table 4.3 (page 76) summarizes the phases of drug testing in the United States.

It is important to clearly understand the possible risks and benefits of participating in clinical drug trials. These risks and benefits must be fully explained in writing before your loved one with AD volunteers to enroll as a participant. All human studies of experimental drugs at reputable medical research centers in cooperation with pharmaceutical companies and government agencies have built-in safeguards. Participation in these studies involves no financial cost, and the risk of harm is minimal due to the ethical standards and strict protocols followed.

Table 4.3: Phases of Testing New Drugs in Humans

	Phase One	Phase Two	Phase Three
Number of Participants	20–100 healthy volunteers	Up to several hundred volunteers with disease	Up to several thousand volunteers with disease
Length of Time	Up to one year	Up to two years	One to four years
Purpose	Mainly safety	Mainly effectiveness and to determine dosage levels	Safety, effectiveness, and ease of administration

(*Source: Food and Drug Administration*, "From Test Tube to Patient: New Drug Development in the U.S.," Consumer: The Magazine of the Food and Drug Administration 2 [1995].)

A promising drug is first tested for effectiveness and safety using test-tube and animal studies in the laboratory. This preliminary phase may last from one to six years, and if the drug shows enough promise, it moves to the first phase of human testing. This step requires the approval of the FDA. In phase one of human testing, the drug is tested mainly for safety among a small number of people, usually fewer than one hundred healthy volunteers; this phase typically lasts about a year. If the first round is successful, the testing moves to phase two.

In phase two, the drug is tested among several hundred individuals who have the disease the drug is intended to treat; this phase can last up to two years. In this phase researchers employ a method known as a double-blind, placebo-controlled study. Participants are randomly assigned to two groups: One group is given the experimental drug and the other group receives a placebo, a pill without active ingredients. The studies are considered double blind because neither the participants nor the researchers know who is receiving the drug and who is receiving the placebo until after the study has been completed. A third party keeps track of this information to monitor any serious side effects of the drug and to complete an analysis of test results. If phase two is successful, then the next round of clinical trials involves an even greater number of people with the disease, from several hundred to a thousand.

In phase three, the double-blind, placebo-controlled method is again used. This phase may last from one to four years. During phase three, researchers may offer an "open-label" option as an incentive for participation in the study. In an open-label study, all participants who complete the study are given the option of taking the experimental drug for six months to one year before the drug manufacturer applies to the FDA for approval. If the drug proves beneficial and safe by the end of this third phase, then an application is submitted to the FDA for review.

Further testing may be required before the FDA makes a final determination to either approve or deny the new drug application. After careful scrutiny of all information regarding safety and effectiveness collected at all phases of testing, the FDA makes a determination whether the drug should be approved for public use, usually through a doctor's prescription. Even if a drug is approved, the pharmaceutical company is required to continue submitting reports describing the drug's performance. Overall, pharmaceutical companies average about a 20-percent success rate in moving new drugs through the human phases of testing to approval for marketing. The approval process from beginning to end usually takes more than ten years and costs millions of dollars. The high price of new drugs is directly related to the research and development phases.

Much research focuses more on finding answers to basic questions about the nature of the disease, rather than drugs to treat it.

There are studies to identify additional risk factors for AD, different methods of diagnosis, and nonmedical ways of treating mood and behavioral problems, to name but a few. Such research projects may not offer any immediate or personal benefits but may lead to knowledge that has practical applications for others in the future. Altruism is at the heart of participation in this type of research, and people with AD and their families often feel good about their roles as volunteers in this important work. Regardless of outcome, they know that they have done their share to expand knowledge about AD. They are like the builders of the European cathedrals that took decades to complete: Although they may never witness the end result of their contribution, they believe that the combined efforts of many people will some day result in solving the great puzzle of AD.

It should be noted, however, that participating in research is not for everyone. Most studies are strictly controlled, and only people meeting certain criteria may be eligible to participate. Also, some studies may involve risks that may not seem worthwhile to you. Finally, time and energy are needed to participate. To find out about research studies being conducted in your local area, contact one of the federally funded centers listed in the Resources section of this book or your local chapter of the Alzheimer's Association or the Alzheimer Society.

THE LIMITS OF MEDICINE

The underlying causes of AD, as well as potential treatments and means of prevention, are being investigated at research centers throughout the world. As scientists work hard to put together millions of pieces in the AD puzzle, you should not feel compelled to spend precious time and energy looking for a remedy that has eluded countless others. The media regularly report new advances in AD research that may or not have real applications in the long run. For now, understanding the symptoms, diagnosis, treatments, and possible causes is a necessary starting point for families and friends of those with AD. Accurate and updated information on the medical aspects of the disease can be gleaned from a variety of sources—books, newsletters, scientific journals, and the Internet. However, medical knowledge about the disease reveals little about how to best care for someone with the disease. Renowned physician William Osler, M.D., once cautioned fellow physicians and medical students about their priorities in this regard: "Care more for the individual patient than for the special features of the disease."[19] Medical science has relatively little to offer right now in the way of treatment, but there is a lot you can offer in terms of care. Human compassion, skill, and imagination may be far more effective than any drug treatment in enhancing the quality of life of someone with AD.

Scientific studies of AD have little or no value for family members and friends unless they yield practical applications. Unfortunately, how to best care for someone with AD receives sparse attention in most medical circles. Science receives the most attention, and the personal aspect of the disease is not seen as a science. Yet the art of human caring is no less deserving of study than science. Millions of people worldwide are affected daily by this disease. They cannot afford to wait for neuroscientists or pharmaceutical companies to provide solutions for their pressing problems. On a practical level, more funds are needed for research into the causes, treatment, and prevention of the disease. In the meantime, parallel efforts should be made to make life more livable for everyone affected by the disease.

Generally, family members and friends of those with AD are better served by focusing on the everyday concerns of providing care. In the end, the intellectual work involved in learning about the disease is less strenuous than the emotional work involved in caring for someone with the disease. I have devoted the remaining chapters in this book mainly to the human art of caring. In the next chapter, I will focus specifically on how to better understand the changing world of the person with AD.

PART II

~

Giving
Care

CHAPTER 5

What Is It Like to Have Alzheimer's Disease?

What we see depends upon
where we sit.

Ram Dass

Whereas the first part of this book covered the medical aspects of AD, this next part concerns the art of caring for someone with the disease. Even though individuals with AD share many of the same symptoms, their unique personalities, backgrounds, and lifestyles greatly influence the ways in which they respond to their disease. However, the person's past ways of coping with difficulties may not always be evident, due to changes in thinking brought on by the disease. It is therefore crucial for you and others to first understand how the person with AD perceives his or her symptoms, and how they affect his or her daily life. Understanding the individual's perspective can be very useful for you, the family members and friends, in adjusting your expectations to the person's needs.

In this chapter, I focus on how people living with the disease experience it in different ways. To this end, I offer an assortment of personal stories to show just how varied the experience of AD can be.

Unlike the growing body of literature by victims and survivors of diseases such as cancer, there is relatively little material available about the experience of living with AD. Because of the very nature of the disease, people with AD have difficulty remembering and expressing their thoughts and feelings in customary ways. Their self-reflection is limited by forgetfulness. It is not surprising, then, that less than ten books have been authored by people with AD, written with the help of their loved ones.[1] A few other people with AD have shared their thoughts in newspapers, newsletters, television interviews, or educational videotapes. Two quarterly newsletters have recently begun to give a voice to those with the disease, *Early Alzheimer's: A Forum for Early Stage Dementia Care* and *Perspectives: A Newsletter for Individuals Diagnosed with Alzheimer's Disease*.[2] Although these publications regularly include first-person accounts, these reflections do not necessarily represent the full spectrum of opinions about living with the disease.

Only a handful of people among the millions with AD have produced books. This fact suggests that they are probably exceptional individuals with a high degree of awareness about their disease who retained a remarkable ability to communicate. While their insights may offer important clues about the experiences of others with the disease, it would probably be a mistake to expect everyone with AD to have the high degree of insight that these individuals have shown. Still, all of these stories are worth reading since they may give you a better understanding of your loved one's experience and help you cope more effectively.

SOME COMMON EXPERIENCES AND FEELINGS

The personal stories shared in published works by those with AD have some basic themes in common. The authors often describe disturbing feelings of alienation, loneliness, and fear, yet on a positive note, they also convey a deepened appreciation for life's simple pleasures. In *Partial View: An Alzheimer's Journey*, former history professor Cary Henderson describes his sense of alienation from others:

Being dense is a very big part of Alzheimer's. Although I'm not as bad as I sometimes am, it comes and goes. It's a very come-and-go disease. When I make a real blunder, I tend to get defensive about it; I have a sense of shame for not knowing what I should have known. And for not being able to think things and see things that I saw several years ago when I was a normal person—but everybody by this time knows I'm not a normal person, and I'm quite aware of that.[3]

He also tells of his intense loneliness due to his disease: "I think one of the worst things about Alzheimer's disease is that you are so alone with it. Nobody around you really knows what's going on. And half the time, or most of the time, we don't know what's going on ourselves."[4]

Loneliness and alienation also show up as themes in other books written by individuals with AD. In his remarkable book, *My Journey into Alzheimer's Disease*, Robert Davis writes of that alienation:

As soon as my diagnosis was announced, some people became very uncomfortable around me. I realize that the shock and pain are difficult to deal with at first. It was strange that in most cases I had to make the effort to seek out people who were avoiding me and look them in the eye and say, "I don't bite. I am still the same person, but I just can't do my work anymore. I know that one of these days I will not be in here anymore, but for now, I am still home in here and I need your friendship and acceptance."[5]

In his personal account, *Show Me the Way to Go Home*, Larry Rose writes of feeling cut off from the mainstream of life: "I can feel myself sliding down that slippery slope. I have a sadness and anxiety that I have never experienced before. It feels like I am the only person in the world with this disease."[6] He also reports:

I am becoming more and more withdrawn. It is much easier to stay in the safety of my home, where Stella treats me with love and respect, than to expose myself to people who don't understand, people who raise their eyebrows when I have trouble making the right change at the cash register, or when I'm unable to think of the right words when asked a question.

Maybe it would be easier for them if I didn't look so healthy."
He later uses a dark image to express his feelings of isolation:
"I feel that I am walking a precipice alone. No one understands
the frustration in my thoughts."[7]

In *Living in the Labyrinth*, Diana McGowin sums up her emotional distance from others by quoting a haunting line from a
screenplay: "The loneliest thing in the world is to be standing
when everyone is sitting... and they all look at you and ask,
'What is wrong with her?'"[8] In her memoir about living with AD
in the early stages, Christine Boden pleads for understanding as
she describes not feeling "normal" any longer: "But we can't help
the way we are—we know that there is something terribly wrong
with us, and we seem to be losing touch with even who we are. We
need all the help we can get."[9]

Although feelings of alienation and loneliness are often mentioned in these personal accounts, perhaps most troubling are the
experiences of fear. Robert Davis writes, "Perhaps the first spiritual
change I noticed was fear. I have never really known fear before.
At night when it is total blackness, these absurd fears come....
The old emotions are gone as new uncontrolled, fearful emotions
sweep in to replace them."[10] Diana McGowin tells of a recurring
fear that her husband might abandon her: "What would become
of me? I needed his moral support and repeatedly sought his vow
to take care of me for the rest of my life. Upon receiving his assur-
ance once again, I would inquire if he knew just how difficult
keeping it may become in the future."[11] Cary Henderson often
notes that paranoia is central to his experience of AD and adds,
"I guess that the disease does make us kind of irrational. Sometimes it's out of fear and sometimes it's being seemingly left out of
things. But it's hard not to be suspicious and I sure hope that
nobody holds that against me."[12]

Odd though it may seem, a deepened appreciation of simple
pleasures is also a theme amidst these personal stories about feeling alienated, alone, and fearful. According to Robert Davis, "A
journey into Alzheimer's is also a journey into the very basic sim-
plicities of life."[13] In spite of a high degree of awareness of their
symptoms and of the resulting changes in their lifestyles, a positive

adaptation to the disease is evident. For example, Christine Boden notes:

> I am more stretched out somehow, more linear, more step-by-step in my thoughts … I'm like a slow-motion version of my old self—not physically but mentally. It's not all bad, as I have more inner space in this linear mode to listen, to see, to appreciate clouds, leaves, flowers…. I am less driven and less impatient.[14]

Larry Rose writes too about some benefits: "There have been many changes in my life since the onset of Alzheimer's, some of which I am not at all ungrateful for. I have more compassion for people, birds, deer, and the like. I have fallen more and more in love with Stella."[15] Diana McGowin observes that her disease has given her a new perspective: "This knowledge enables me to savor life more openly and ravenously. I appreciate all good things more, whether they be trusted friends, cherished memories, nature's beauty or physical pleasures."[16] The search for something positive in the personal experience of AD is repeated throughout Thaddeus Raushi's remarkably upbeat book, *A View From Within*. Although well aware of his losses due to AD, he prefers instead to adjust his attitude to fit the situation: "It has to do with little things in life elevated to a level of appreciation. It has to do with cherishing relationships."[17] The human capacity for resilience in the face of hardship is striking throughout these personal accounts about living with AD.

Adaptation to AD may seem surprising given the daily frustrations imposed by the disease and its relentless nature. The awareness of decline in mental abilities is often coupled with appreciation of the remaining gifts in one's life. Those who find some peace in the midst of their confusion tend to challenge our assumptions about what it might feel like to live with the disease. Former President Ronald Reagan's letter to the American public in late 1994 also illustrates this important point. He expresses concern about what the future may hold for his wife, yet the overall tone of his letter is not pessimistic. On the contrary, Mr. Reagan writes of his intention to continue enjoying outdoor activities and to stay in touch with friends and supporters. He ends his letter by noting, "I now begin the journey into the sunset of my life."[18] This metaphor may jar our expectations about what he should be thinking or saying about having AD. Shouldn't he feel angry or sad? Is he merely in a state of denial? Is he just putting the expected political spin on a bad situation? How can the man once considered the most politically powerful person in the world calmly face this state of powerlessness? After all, wouldn't I feel awful if I had just been told I have AD? Like many people with AD, who because of their decreased ability to intellectualize no longer hide their true feelings, Mr. Reagan was probably simply expressing that yesterday and tomorrow are no longer priorities and that he has confidence that others will attend to details as he proceeds on his "journey."

In a newsletter of the Los Angeles chapter of the Alzheimer's Association, a relative of someone with AD criticizes Mr. Reagan for his viewpoint: "He errs when he calls it 'the journey into the sunset of my life.' His words make it sound like a pleasant twilight stroll. In truth, it's a terrifying plunge into the void of midnight."[19] This criticism may represent the perspectives of some family members who bear witness to profound changes in their loved ones; however, it does not take into account that personal experience of the disease is as unique as the individuals who have it. It is perhaps unfair to judge Mr. Reagan or others whose subjective experience of AD differs from what we know, or assume to know, about a person with the disease.

To understand the state of mind of someone with AD, it is necessary to reexamine our expectations of how he or she should think or feel. To relieve the person with AD of the pressure to think or act "normally," we must accept the current reality of the individual—no matter how distorted it may seem. Trying to force people with AD into our version of reality does them a disservice and lowers their self-esteem by emphasizing their limitations instead of their remaining strengths. People with AD simply cannot keep pace with our old expectations, and under the circumstances we must adopt new ones that will accommodate the demands of the disease. Ethicist Stephen Post stresses the need to reconsider our point of view:

Because our culture so values rationality and productivity, observers easily characterize the life of persons with dementia in the bleakest terms.... The experience of the person with irreversible and progressive dementia is clearly tragic, but it need not be interpreted as half empty rather than as half full.[20]

Cary Henderson puts this sentiment in a uniquely personal way: "There are things that I wish I could do, but on the other side, there are still things that I can still do and I plan to hold on to them as long as I possibly can."[21] Likewise, Charlton Heston eloquently conveyed his fighting spirit when he announced in August 2002 that he had been diagnosed with AD: "I'm neither giving up nor giving in.... I must reconcile courage and surrender in equal measure. Please feel no sympathy for me. I don't. I just may be a little less accessible to you, despite my wishes."[22]

VARYING DEGREES OF AWARENESS OF SYMPTOMS

At one time, it was assumed that everyone with AD was unaware of their memory loss and not troubled by it. Even today, some medical professionals mistakenly believe this to be true in all cases. Some people, such as those quoted above, are quite aware of their symptoms, while others seem oblivious of them. Still others with the disease fluctuate in their awareness, quite aware if they are taxed beyond their abilities but unaware if they are not challenged. For the most part, people with AD have a partial or limited insight into how the disease affects their lives. The disease often diminishes awareness about the nature and severity of symptoms, as if a dimmer switch has been lowered that reduces the ability to see things clearly.

No one is sure what accounts for these differing levels of awareness. Personality may play a role, but does not alone account for such range of experiences. The extent and location of damage to the brain may also influence a person's degree of insight. Growing evidence, based on brain-imaging studies, shows that the level of awareness is linked to the deterioration of the frontal lobe, the part of the brain associated with awareness, insight, and judgment. As AD advances over time, personal awareness of one's symptoms generally diminishes too—a strange sort of blessing.

How people with AD perceive their symptoms is key to understanding how they might receive your help. There is a good chance that someone who recognizes the limitations and effects of AD will see your help as necessary. Someone who is unaware of their symptoms may see your helpful efforts as unnecessary, demeaning, and intrusive. A trusting relationship with the person who has AD can enhance the level of cooperation, but trust alone will not win over someone who cannot see the need for help. Even though you have the best of intentions, you may not be able to persuade someone to accept your assistance.

For the minority of people with AD who are acutely aware of their disease, daily life can be quite frustrating, as the above quoted authors illustrate. They may feel self-conscious and worry about making mistakes. Although they often try to compensate for or cover up their lapses, their efforts may fall short of their own expectations or those of others. They may become seriously depressed if they dwell on their failures, blame themselves for the problems caused by the disease, or say they feel stupid or make other self-deprecating remarks.

People with AD who are aware of their limitations may also take out their frustrations on loved ones. For example, in an article in the *Chicago Sun-Times,* Donald Baron, who has AD, writes about his displeasure with his wife's changing role in their marriage: "I get very angry with my wife, Jean. She's always bossing me around, telling me what I can do, what I can't do."[23] Likewise, in a videotaped interview, Dr. David Bronson reveals his misplaced anger about having the disease: "I'm not in charge. I'm not free to come and go as I've done in the past. I feel frequently that my wife thinks she owns me now. I guess part of my anger is being directed toward her when she is trying to fill in the gaps for me. I feel that I'm not my own person anymore."[24]

In contrast, many people with AD express gratitude for the help of others. Noting his pride in his wife, one man told me:

I'd like to get my memory better, but there's not much that can be done about it. I just do the best I can. My wife watches me like a hawk. Whatever has to be done, she'll say, 'Joe, I'll do it or I'll help you do it.' I get plenty of help. I know what she's doing. I've got the greatest wife in the world.

In an Alzheimer's Association newsletter article, Gloria Sterin credits her husband's tact in helping her to cope: "He is my bulwark. The best thing about him is that he is willing to let me do as much as I can by myself. He does not hover over me and tell me I can't do things. Instead, he offers support and encouragement. I never feel inadequate when he's around."[25]

Clearly, those who are aware of their disease vary in their response to living with its effects. Some are conflicted about asking for or receiving help. One woman with AD interviewed for the *Perspectives* newsletter expresses mixed feelings: "I fought like hell—every single step—in getting help. I'd think, 'I don't need it yet or I don't want it now.' Then eventually I'd think, 'I really do need help now. It won't hurt me.' I'm always glad when I do get help. It's a slow process, I guess."[26] This struggle between independence and dependence will be discussed again in the next chapter.

At the other end of the spectrum are those who appear completely oblivious to their disease. Sometimes they are described as being in a state of denial, a common defense mechanism that shields the human psyche from painful realities. However, this description is generally not useful in understanding people with the disease. Faulty memory and judgment, not denial, lead many people with AD to believe that they are intact. They may not realize that they are forgetting names or places, or may not be troubled by it. To put it simply, they forget that they forget. As a result, their frustration may be mild, even nonexistent. They firmly believe that all is well. Their egos, built on a lifetime of achievements, remain so well preserved that they cannot recognize what is apparent to others. For example, James Anthony made this observation in describing the trouble he had performing his job due to AD: "I was not aware that I was having difficulties, but my difficulties were made plain when my supervisor pointed out my lapses in a very abrasive manner.... You cannot experience what you have forgotten."[27] Therefore, confronting people who are oblivious about their impairments is not only pointless, but also may be upsetting for all concerned. The disease is to blame for their seeming lack of concern. Since they are unaware of the need for help, it is very difficult to elicit their cooperation, even when help is clearly needed.

The following excerpts from interviews I conducted with various people with AD further illustrate this lack of awareness.

An eighty-year-old retired railroad worker reports: "I'm slower than I was because I'm older. My wife says my memory is real bad, but I don't notice it." He goes on to explain, "I can do anything I always did. Maybe not as fast but I do it. I still drive a car! My wife says I forget where I'm going but I don't think so. She gets mad at me because I forget. She says that I don't do anything. She says I should be more active. It bothers her more than it bothers me."

A seventy-year-old homemaker explains, "I don't believe I have a memory problem because I have a better memory than the average person. I mean this sincerely. In fact, I have a better memory than my husband." About the impact of AD on her life, she notes, "I do the same things I did all the time. I wash, I cook, I iron, and I shop. I try to manage as much as I can. I can forget things, but you know, I'm not a youngster anymore."

Writing for an Alzheimer's Association newsletter, James Anthony leaves room for the role of denial in his experience of AD and suggests that some degree of denial is useful:

> Remarkably, a number of us with Alzheimer's are chipper. I'm not sure why. My guess is that having gotten the heavy news, we decide we will make the most of being with friends and family, and of doing things we love to do. It's a prescription that people without Alzheimer's might try. I do not mean to suggest that people with Alzheimer's do not take the measure of our prospects . . . [but] a degree of denial is essential. Like somebody drinking hot coffee, we sip the truth of our condition carefully and gently.[28]

In general, people who are either highly aware of their disease or completely oblivious to it are a minority of those with AD.[29] For most people in the early stages, personal awareness fluctuates but generally remains at a lower level than expected, as insight into the nature and degree of their impairments is blunted by the disease. Most people don't dwell on their impairments, or they find ways to excuse them.

The following interview excerpts illustrate the partial or low level of awareness that is fairly common among those in the early stages of the disease.

A seventy-five-year-old retired electrician reports, "I've got memory problems. I'm not so sharp the way I used to be. I guess old age is creeping in, so we've got to take it whether we like it or not. A lot of people are worse off than I am, so I have to take it one day at a time and hope for the best." He later says:

> I still don't see much difference in my life, you know. I worked as an electrician in a shop so I always used my hands. I was pretty good too. I'm still busy all the time. I got my home and my garden and I'm always fiddling around. I always find a job to do. I do what I'm familiar with and if I'm asked to do something different, I can ask for advice.

A seventy-three-year-old retired teacher comments:

> I've read about this disease. I don't have as much use for my memory as I used to. You see, the things I forget are the things I don't come in contact with anymore, I would say. If I forget, I either look it up or ask my husband, because we're both at home. I'll say, "Honey, I forgot this and that. Can you remember?" And he will help me remember.

Regarding her expectations for the future, she notes, "Well, I just hope that my health lasts the way it has. I hope I can live the way I am now in spirit and body, because I have a very good life."

Because of their inability to recall the recent past or plan ahead for the future, people with AD naturally tend to focus on the present and the distant past. Although cognizant of losses or changes, they often begin a gradual process of adaptation to their disease. Over time, people with AD generally lower their expectations of their own abilities, instead of struggling to maintain former standards of thinking and doing things. As one woman observes, "My mother knows that she doesn't remember and knows that she can't do certain things on her own. She takes it very calmly. It doesn't frustrate her the way it would frustrate me." As the recent past and future dwindle in importance, and other people assume responsibility for remembering and planning for them, affected people can experience the "here and now" more freely. The experience of living in the present moment takes on a deeper meaning. In a newsletter article, Jan Soukop recounts an incident that enabled her to appreciate the present moment. After describing her mourning over "the loss of what was and what might be," she notes:

> One day as I fumbled around the kitchen to make a pot of coffee, something caught my eye through the window. It had snowed and I had forgotten what a beautiful sight a soft, gentle snowfall could be. I eagerly dressed and went outside to join my son who was shoveling our driveway. As I bent down to gather a mass of those radiantly white flakes on my shovel, it seemed as though I could do nothing but marvel at their beauty. Needless to say, my son did not share in my enthusiasm. To him it was nothing more than a job; but to me it was an experience. Later, I realized that for a short period of time, God granted me the ability to see snowfall through the same innocent eyes of the child I once was, so many years ago. Jan is still there I thought, and there will be wonders to behold in each new day. They will just be different now.[30]

Clearly, how people with AD perceive their symptoms is highly individualized and may be radically different from our image of what it might feel like to us. Furthermore, in trying to understand the thinking and behavior of people with AD, we can no longer simply rely on our past experiences with them. In fact, past experience may actually limit our insight into how the affected person is being challenged by the disease. This suggests that, no matter how compassionate or empathetic we may be, when we try to understand the thoughts and feelings of those with AD, there is a chance that our assumptions may be mistaken. A whole new way of thinking and acting is usually required to accommodate the changing perceptions of someone with AD.

THE IMPORTANCE OF SOCIAL
ENVIRONMENT

Anyone who has ever become disabled, regardless of the underlying condition, experiences a sense of losing her or his place in the world. For people with AD this is true in both literal and figurative terms, since becoming disoriented about time and place is a common symptom. On another level, one's sense of self may feel threatened as connections to other people, places, and things start to slip over time. The world can easily become a confusing place. Therefore, it is vital for people with AD to have caring people who can help connect them to their environment. In fact, the presence or absence of caring people may be the most significant factor in determining the quality of life for someone with AD.

This feeling of becoming unmoored or disoriented was described in Dr. Alzheimer's original case report of a middle-aged woman with AD. This unfortunate woman, now known by the name of Auguste D., was uprooted from her family and home in 1901 and placed in a psychiatric hospital in Frankfurt, Germany, until her death in 1905. According to Dr. Alzheimer's written notes, she often remarked, "I have lost myself."[31] Although her disease had caused her disorientation, the stark surroundings in which she was forced to live most likely intensified it. There was little or nothing to keep her feeling connected to her past life. No familiar experiences were provided to rekindle her interest and satisfaction in everyday life. In the abnormal lifestyle of the hospital, cut off from familiar people and activities, it was no wonder that Auguste D. experienced a loss of self. Her diminished coping skills due to the disease, combined with an impoverished environment, must have made her life miserable.

Although it has been nearly a century since Dr. Alzheimer encountered Auguste D., the importance of helping those with AD to feel connected to the world and other people is still not completely understood. At one time it was believed that an individual's life before the onset of the disease had little or no bearing on his or her experience of AD. Moreover, it was believed that nothing could influence the progressive course of the disease and that quality of life would be marginal at best. In recent years, these assumptions have been challenged by the growing realization that much can be done to enhance the well-being of people with AD.

Some researchers have suggested that when family and friends compensate for the disabilities of the person with AD and promote remaining abilities, the rate of decline may be slowed.[32] Just as an impoverished environment can intensify people's symptoms and diminish their quality of life, an enriched environment may positively influence their disease process and improve their quality of life. This requires great sensitivity about their physical, psychological, and social needs and taking responsibility for meeting those needs. Rather than relying exclusively on medical treatments to improve the well-being of those with AD, we can instead focus on our personal interactions with them, which can often do far more to influence their quality of life. A good relationship is better than the most powerful drug.

WHAT DO PEOPLE WITH AD
REALLY NEED?

Although every person with AD is unique, and individual preferences must be respected, people with the disease generally share the same basic needs. In addition to the physical need for food, clothing, and shelter, people with AD require three other things to be relatively happy: intimacy, community, and meaningful activity.

Intimacy refers to closeness to and familiarity with other people, places, and things. In an intimate relationship such as a marriage or friendship, individuals care about one another and look out for one another's welfare. Without intimacy, fear and loneliness prevail. When the need for intimacy is not met, a host of real and imagined fears commonly take root in people with AD. They may fear losing control of their life or being abandoned by family and friends. One man noted that his wife with AD became obsessed with locking the doors to their home because she was worried about intruders. A woman with AD told me one day, "I worry that my husband is having an affair and will leave me." They may fear becoming dependent and becoming a burden to others. A man with AD expressed frustration about his reliance on his daughter: "The thing I hate the most is always asking her for reminders. She's got better things to do than looking after me. She's got a life of her own, after all." Whether or not these worries are warranted, they are quite real to the person with AD. Intimacy through physical touch, as well as staying in touch with others, helps someone with AD to overcome these fears.

Sometimes this need for intimacy is exaggerated, as seen in those who cling to or "shadow" their loved ones. Just being in the physical presence of a trusted person at all times may offer reassurance to someone with AD who otherwise feels fearful while alone or with strangers. Likewise, feeling connected to a familiar and safe place such as one's home can also be comforting. Again, this may be exaggerated in the form of the person with AD resisting invitations to go outside the home. Even closeness with pets or other favorite things can offer comfort. Cary Henderson's personal account includes much praise for his dog, including a suggestion for others with AD: "I sort of think that anybody with Alzheimer's could benefit by a friendly little dog. Somebody they can play with and talk to—it's kinda nice to talk to a dog that you know is not going to talk back. And you cannot make a mistake that way."[33] Larry Rose's story of living with AD, Show Me the Way to Go Home, is also filled with funny and touching references to his constant companion, a pot-bellied pig named Floyd.

People with AD need intimacy perhaps more than ever. As they gradually lose their customary ways of connecting with other people and the world, they need others to reach out to them and help them feel connected. And because their sense of initiative often wanes, others must extend themselves to meet this need for intimacy in active ways. Intimate relationships make people with AD feel safe and allow them to enjoy being known and appreciated.

Community refers to a sense of belonging to a group with whom one shares a common bond. This community can consist of just one other person, a family, or a larger group of people who can see beyond superficial realities to the value of each person. People with AD may feel cut off from their family, friends, and neighbors due to their forgetfulness and other impairments. Like the lepers of biblical times, they often feel rejected, unwelcome, or out of place in a society that places a high value on self-reliance, productivity, and intellectual prowess. People with AD often think and act differently from those who are considered "normal." They may feel alienated and embarrassed when they fail to remember names or cannot complete a simple task. A man with AD admitted to me: "I used to be full of self-confidence, but now I'm quite conscious of making mistakes. I do not want to appear foolish in front of other people." A true community, however, recognizes the diversity of human experiences and allows everyone to be treated in humane and dignified ways—especially those who have a disability.

People with AD need reassurance that they are accepted for who they are and not for what they can do. Belonging to a caring community means that someone with AD is accepted without the usual conditions being met. Their limitations are downplayed, while their remaining strengths are celebrated. The personal worth of someone with AD can be sustained if others share this vision of a caring and inclusive community. Family members and friends can learn to create this warm and friendly atmosphere, and thereby enrich the lives of everyone involved. The need for community is often met in support groups for people with AD by virtue of their shared concerns. One woman with AD praised her support group, saying, "I am at peace when I'm with my group. I can be myself without pretending that I am a hundred percent. The group has been my lifeline. Everyone there understands what it feels like to be lost and forgetful. It makes no difference to us."

Finally, people with AD need to be involved in *meaningful activities*. Preconceived notions about productive work or hobbies must be replaced with new ideas for activities that suit their abilities and disabilities. If placed in a situation where they can do little or nothing for themselves, they will feel inadequate and slip into passivity. But if given opportunities for active participation, no matter how small their role may be, affirmation and success are possible.

Activities are the everyday stuff of life. Cooking a meal, making a bed, cleaning a room, singing a tune, shopping for food, caring for a pet, and taking a walk are the kind of informal activities that can give life meaning for the person with AD. Such ordinary things can highlight a person's remaining abilities and create opportunities to give to others instead of always being the recipient of care. People with AD can do some of these activities alone, but more often they need the encouragement and support of other people. Consequently, intimacy and community are reinforced through engaging in meaningful activities together. Christine Boden sums up this perspective in her personal account of living with AD: "I want to carry on drinking in the beauty of this world and feel the love of my family and friends. Even if I might not remember these experiences very long, I still want to have them. Surely remembering an experience doesn't constitute the sole enjoyment of that moment!"[34]

People with AD depend on other people to see the world through their eyes and ensure that their needs for intimacy, community, and meaningful activity are met. They need at least one caring person to step forward to serve in the role of a companion, mentor, leader, coach, or best friend. One individual often assumes the primary responsibility of seeing that these needs are met. The fact that you are reading this book suggests that you may be the primary person in this role. In the next chapter I will address how you can best serve your loved one with AD in your role as a "leader."

WHAT SOME FAMILY MEMBERS HAVE TO SAY

The following quotes from relatives of people with AD illustrate how caring and compassionate relationships are at the heart of meeting needs. More advice from relatives of people with AD will be shared in Chapter 13.

Geri comments about her mother with AD:

> She needs for us to say, "It's okay to be like this, Mom. We still like you. People still want to be with you." We have to give her

a push to get back into society or she would stay home all of the time. We make sure that she eats and her clothes are clean. We try to make sure she does things for herself too.

Marge makes this observation about her husband with AD: "He needs me to be in charge. If that appears difficult for me, he feels guilty that he is a burden to me. He needs to know that I'm okay with this and that I'm in it for the long haul."

George offers this assessment of his wife: "More than anything else, she needs to be kept happy. I don't want her to be in any situation where she is befuddled. I look out for her and for myself as well."

Fred simply notes about his wife: "She needs for me to keep cool. If I get upset, so does she."

Mary says this about her husband:

He needs my love and affection. He needs direction too. He will do anything I ask of him but he will not volunteer to do anything. I told him today to go to the local gas station to get the gas can filled for the lawnmower and to pick up a newspaper too. He got the newspaper but forgot about the gas can. I should have known better.

Frank says this about his sister: "It isn't the practical help so much as the moral support. I would never think of harping on her because she cannot remember a name. If she wants to tell a story but can't remember the names of the people involved, I tell her to go ahead anyway."

Phillip notes, "My mother always wants to be busy. She lives alone and if she is by herself for more than a day, she is not happy. She needs my time and support."

Sally describes her approach with her husband:

He needs gentle reminders. I try to make light of it. I know he needs lots of love and praise from me. I leave him alone unless I know he's really struggling with something. If I jump in too fast, he gets aggravated. I would rather have him succeed on his own and feel good about his accomplishments.

These family members did not come to a sudden understanding of their unique position in the life of a loved one with AD. Rather, with time and experience, they gradually adjusted to their new role. This process required a profound shift in how they viewed their relationship with the individual who was changing due to the disease. They slowly learned how to make changes to fit the situation. In the next chapter I will address many of the important aspects of these changing roles and responsibilities.

CHAPTER 6

. . . .
                .
                .
                .

How Relationships, Roles, and Responsibilities Change

*Since we cannot change reality,
let us change the eyes which see
reality.*

Nikos Kazantzakis

Alzheimer's disease inevitably leads to changes in relationships. Similar to the progression of the disease, these changes are subtle at first but slowly become profound. People with AD can no longer function as they once did. Their communication and reasoning skills gradually falter. They can no longer handle alone responsibilities that they once took for granted. As a result, you must learn to accept your loved one's declining abilities and make adjustments. Your relationship with the affected person cannot continue as it once was. You will have to change your expectations of what she or he can and cannot do independently, compensate for the disabilities, and assume a growing number of responsibilities. As one woman said about her husband with AD, "We are the ones who must change. He cannot and will not change to suit us."

In this chapter, I discuss your unique role in the life of the person with AD as well as the changing nature of your relationship with relatives, friends, and others. If your spouse or long-term partner has AD, the sad truth is that your relationship will never be the same again. You will need to assume a more active role in your relationship than ever before. If your mother or father has AD, your relationship with your parent will also change. The time and energy that you will need to devote to various things formerly done by your parent will increase over time. And your involvement with a spouse or parent who has AD will probably affect all your other relationships as well—with loved ones at home, with siblings, with friends, and with coworkers.

ACCEPTING THE DIAGNOSIS

The first step is to accept that the diagnosis of AD is a permanent reality. It is natural in the beginning to want to deny this—denial is the human psyche's way of protecting us from feeling the terrible effects of painful situations. It allows time for the news to sink in. You may initially dismiss the symptoms of AD in your loved one until something forces the issue of getting a diagnosis. You may doubt the diagnosis, and seek a second or third opinion. This is understandable and completely normal. Doubt initially enables you to prepare emotionally for the reality and the practical implications of living with the disease. Keep this in mind as you deal with others who may have difficulty accepting the news or who doubt the seriousness of the situation.

Denial is often reinforced by the misleading—or seemingly absent—symptoms of the disease. After all, the person with AD may appear physically healthy. One man commented about his wife, "Because she looks as good as she does, it's really hard to believe that her brain is really sick." A daughter noted, "It's easy to overlook my mother's need for help. She looks just fine, in spite of her difficulties. In fact, she looks much better than the average person her age. It's tempting to forget that she really has Alzheimer's."

The fluctuating nature of the symptoms can also make you wonder about the diagnosis. There may be days when the person with AD is like his or her old self much of the time. So many faculties may be intact that you may be led to minimize or disregard the person's impairments. Gloria Hoffman speaks to this point in the educational video, *Caring About Howard:* "There was a time that I was on such a roller coaster. He'd be real good one day and I'd think, 'Is there anything wrong with him?' And then the next day, he couldn't remember anything. One day I'd be elated and then the next day I'd be down."[1] One husband confided to me:

> Even though she was diagnosed with Alzheimer's a year ago, I keep having this internal argument about whether she has this disease. Upon the recommendation of a therapist, I have started telling myself once a day, "Yes, she does have Alzheimer's disease." Saying this seems to be helping to quiet my mind.

Your reluctance to accept the diagnosis may be reinforced by the person with AD, who could be adamant about holding on to personal freedom and autonomy. Values of self-reliance and individualism are deeply rooted in our culture. We seldom, if ever, wish to appear dependent on others for anything. Men in particular have traditionally associated dependence with personal weakness and a threat to their masculinity. And women, who have traditionally been responsible for caring for others, may resist being cared for themselves. One woman with AD explained this dilemma by saying, "When you have always been a person who likes to give assistance, it's hard to be on the receiving end."

Because of these negative connotations of dependence, it is understandable that people with AD may be reticent to ask for help or may resist helpful overtures. Some people with AD express this desire for independence in the form of resentment or hostility toward those who are offering help. At times, there may be an apparent contradiction between their desire for independence and their need to be helped with certain things. The person with AD may give mixed signals: wanting help, wanting to be independent, wanting to be accommodated, or wanting to be treated normally. One man with the disease articulated this inner struggle when he told me, "The strange thing about living with this disease is that you've got to fight it and accept it at the same time."

You should not expect to take in the fullness of the implications of the disease immediately. Understanding—and acceptance—usually occurs in fits and starts. You may feel that you have little or no time in your life for the demands of the disease. Other priorities may take precedence over or compete with the needs of the person with AD. However, you and the affected person will be better off in the long run if you begin now to assume a leadership role in your relationship. The person with AD may suffer adverse consequences if you do not take into account how the disease is disrupting his or her life. By accepting the diagnosis and its life-changing effects, your ability to control your reactions to disease-related changes will improve significantly. The person with the disease will also benefit from your enlightened perspective. You will begin, in a sense, to make room for the disease without letting it completely dominate your life. Try not to feel overwhelmed by the current challenges or those that lie ahead. Time allows for plenty of on-the-job training in learning how to care for someone with AD.

STEPPING INTO THE LEADERSHIP ROLE

Since the person with AD no longer possesses the mental skills to be completely independent, a special brand of leadership is called for. At least one person must assume overall authority for ensuring the well-being of the person with AD, but it is best to include others too, if at all possible. Much work is involved in addressing basic physical needs like food and shelter as well as the psychological and social needs discussed in the previous chapter. You need not be afraid of taking on this important leadership role or a major part of it, although it may feel awkward at first. The person with AD needs your help. If possible, it is best to share this role with someone else or at least to delegate some of the responsibilities to others who are willing to help and support your efforts.

Whether the person with AD is your spouse, parent, sibling, or in-law, a shift in the balance of power must occur in your relationship. You may feel uncomfortable at first with the term "power." Yet the dynamics of power, influence, and authority exist in every relationship and can be used constructively. The change in power balance derives from the fact that the person with AD needs protection from the risks posed by the disease and can no longer meet her or his needs alone. Because of impairment in memory, thinking, or other brain functions, the person with AD no longer has intellectual equality with others—an unfortunate reality. As one person's role in the relationship changes and personal control diminishes, the other person's role must change in corresponding ways.

Any person giving direction and assuming greater responsibility in a relationship is exercising more power than the other person. This does not mean, however, that the dignity of the person with AD should be diminished or ignored. On the contrary, preserving his or her dignity becomes the utmost priority. In taking leadership, your job is not to dominate the life of the person with AD, but to help minimize the affected person's disabilities and maximize his or her remaining abilities. This implies not only caring *for* the person with AD but also caring *about* the person. Ultimately, the leadership role is about meeting the needs of the other person.

It takes self-confidence to assume leadership on behalf of another adult. It also takes extraordinary empathy, patience, and understanding to exercise this powerful role in a loving way. Despite the inequality of the relationship, the self-esteem of the person with AD must be upheld. Otherwise, feelings of embarrassment, depression, and frustration may arise, and conflicts may develop. In *Counting on Kindness: The Dilemmas of Dependency,* Wendy Lustbader describes the finesse required of the leader:

> The best assistance is that which is unobtrusive. Helpers who quietly get things done, rather than announcing their efforts, leave a dependent person's pride intact. The indebtedness position is not emphasized, and no mention is made of special accommodations. The fact of helplessness then recedes into the background, where it can reside without harming the person's self-esteem.[2]

Sensitivity to the feelings of the person being helped can lead to mutual understanding and cooperation.

Knowing how and when to help out completely, partially, or not at all also requires you to think on your feet. Sometimes it may seem more efficient for you to take over a task completely. At the same time, by doing so you may be ignoring the remaining abilities of someone with AD. You may reason, "I can fix a meal in half the time it takes him so I might as well do it by myself," even though the person with AD may derive satisfaction from playing a part in meal preparation. At the other extreme, you may assume that a certain task can be done independently, causing the person with AD to struggle needlessly. You may think, "She can still manage paying those bills by herself" when, in fact, she may silently wish for relief from this stressful work. Understanding the different levels of dependence and independence requires much insight into the needs and preferences of the affected person. At the same time, you cannot overlook the limits on your own time, energy, and patience. Balancing all these practical and personal needs can be a real juggling act.

A good metaphor for the changing relationship between you and the person with AD is the relationship between two ballroom dancers. When a couple dances, the roles of leader and follower are carefully orchestrated. A good leader dances in a way that enables the follower to be led almost effortlessly. The leader's cues may be so subtle that the follower may not appear to be led at all. The couple dances together gracefully as each partner cooperates in playing his or her part. In your relationship with a person with AD, you may be called on to change roles from follower to leader.

Another thing about your relationship is that you can no longer take for granted that the person with AD will remember the proper steps. You must now take a more active role in the dance. You must learn when to step in and when to step back. Fluctuations in symptoms will often make it hard for you to gauge when to step in to offer help and when to step back and refrain from helping. In a newspaper article, Jean Baron describes this problem in relation to her husband with AD: "Perhaps hardest is the contradiction between his need for independence and his need for help with some things. This leads him to accuse me, on the one hand, of treating him like a child and, on the other, of not being sensitive to his needs."[3]

It may take a long time—months or even years—for you to learn a new set of "mental gymnastics," even though you may know that a different way of relating is now required. The transition to your new leadership role can evolve over time. In its early stages, the disease does not require that you assume a full-time position as a provider of care. On a practical and emotional level, it is important to keep in mind the limits of your leadership role at this stage. One man shared his thoughts with me about his limited but central role during the early stage of his wife's disease:

> I purposely don't think of myself as a "caregiver," as the word implies a total dependence on her part. This may be a matter of semantics, but I try to differentiate between what she needs for me to do for her and what she can do for herself. So far, the latter far outweighs the former. When that switch takes place, I guess I will have become a caregiver.

Fortunately, since AD progresses very slowly, in most cases you can make the shift in your role as leader bit by bit. The sooner the shift in roles takes place, however, the better it will be for the person with AD. If you are assertive without being domineering, helpful without being overbearing, and kind without being patronizing, then the person with the disease is likely to respond positively to your good intentions.

WHEN YOUR PARTNER HAS AD

If your spouse or long-term partner has AD, how will your new role as leader affect your relationship? The answer to this question may well depend on how you worked out the terms of your relationship in the past. On the one hand, if you tended to be more the leader in the past, then you may possess the experience and self-confidence to assume the responsibilities that your loved one with AD once managed. On the other hand, if the person with AD was more the leader in your relationship, then you are more likely to have difficulty adjusting to the leadership role. Dick

Tilleli, who has AD, writes about the changing roles in his marriage:

> There are times when I have a difficult time doing things, and I ask for her help. I guess that's different from what it used to be. Years ago, I was the macho man. I was the guy who did everything. Now she does most things, and that I don't like. But it's something that has to be done....Most of the time she's right, but sometimes I just want to do what I want to do.[4]

If you and your partner were more or less equals in the past, then you are probably better prepared to accept the changes occurring now.

Likewise, if you have enjoyed a long and happy relationship, your history together may empower you to deal with present and future challenges. However, even the longest unions, lasting fifty or sixty years, are tested by AD. If you had a turbulent marriage, for example, then you may dread caring for a spouse with the disease. On the other hand, if you remarried late in life and didn't have many years together before your spouse got the disease, then you may wonder if you have the commitment to continue in the relationship. In addition, your spouse's children by a former marriage may not readily accept your leadership role. Anything less than a strong relationship may be threatened by the demands imposed by the disease. Mixed feelings are bound to arise.

In committed relationships there is an expectation that each person will do his or her part to nurture the other person. Mutuality and reciprocity are inherent aspects of the marriage agreement or long-term partnership. Unfortunately, AD no longer allows the spouse or long-term partner with the disease to fulfill his or her part of the nurturing bargain. This is often a sad and painful reality for the well spouse, whose partner can no longer participate fully in the marriage or make decisions in traditional ways. While new ways of communicating, solving problems, and expressing love can be discovered, the burden of breaking old habits and creating new ones falls on the shoulders of the well partner. Someone with AD who was your friend, helper, advisor, and intimate companion may no longer be capable of continuing in these roles. And you will no longer be able to take for granted the practical tasks formerly carried out by your partner. You will now need to assume those responsibilities or delegate them to someone else. The following are some examples of this dynamic:

A husband noticed that his wife could no longer prepare hot meals safely and needed supervision: "I had never cooked a meal in our fifty-two years of marriage. Now I'm the chief cook."

A wife realized that her husband could no longer manage their finances: "He resented my help at first. I did not have the skills or experience to deal with brokers, but I eventually caught on. I did not even know how to balance a checkbook until I learned that he was making a mess of things."

A husband said, "It may sound funny, but I did not know how to operate the washing machine. When my wife could no longer do this job, I had to ask my daughter how to do the laundry."

A wife said, "He did all of the grocery shopping after he retired. Then he began to forget items at the store, so I had to resume this responsibility."

After a wife observed her husband's erratic driving, she said, "He had always been the main driver until I realized that he was endangering himself and others. Now I have taken over as the full-time driver, in spite of his resistance."

New or increased responsibilities for such practical tasks are a major part of the changes in the marital relationship. However, expressions of intimacy, including sex, are likely to change too. Intimacy rests on many interconnected abilities that are impaired by AD. These include the capacity to convey one's thoughts and feelings and to comprehend verbal and nonverbal communication. The overall quality of the relationship suffers when the partner with AD can no longer give or receive intimacy in his or her usual way.[5] Furthermore, for reasons not fully understood, sexual interest and function often wane among people with AD. Sexual desire in the healthy partner may also diminish, because of the many changes taking place in the relationship.

Couples who continue to find satisfaction in their relationship, sexual and otherwise, usually do so by redefining the terms of their commitment. Instead of expecting a fifty-fifty partnership, the well partner typically accepts the other partner's limitations and creates new opportunities for shared meaning and closeness. Healthy relationships grow from the flexibility of both partners in responding to changing circumstances in the course of their life together. Although the person with AD may no longer have the capacity to make adjustments, the other partner can, in effect, take the lead in renegotiating their commitment, so that both feel comfortable with their changing roles and responsibilities.

Many committed people who are not married are affected in similar ways when one partner develops AD. For a variety of reasons, a growing number of older people choose to live together without getting married. They may meet late in life after the death of a spouse or a divorce and may decide to live together, but may not wish to formalize their commitment in a marriage. Such partners may have a moral obligation to each other, but they often lack the legal and financial protections afforded to married couples. Likewise, older gay and lesbian couples may have a long-term relationship but without the same rights as married couples. Furthermore, most same-sex couples have paid a high emotional price for their sexual orientation. Their extended families are often split over their lifestyle and over accepting their life-long partner. However, partners in such relationships confront issues similar to those faced by married couples when one partner has AD. The changes that take place in the relationship are equally challenging. Thus, these couples may need to clarify their legal, financial, and social rights to effectively carry out their changing roles and responsibilities in relation to the partner with AD.

WHEN YOUR PARENT HAS AD

If your mother or father has AD, it is natural for you to want to remain in your traditional role as son or daughter. It is difficult to change patterns of behavior with someone you have known your entire life. Expectations and ways of communicating tend to become entrenched in long-lasting relationships—for better or for worse. For example, it may feel odd to act as the decision-maker for someone who had authority over you at one time. But unsettling as it may be at first, impairment in your parent's memory, judgment, language, orientation, and visual-spatial relations will require that you regularly give them direction, reminders, and other forms of help.

If your parent is widowed or divorced, you may be the one who ultimately assumes the leadership role. Does this mean that you are now in a position of "parenting your parent"? It is hard to avoid thinking of being in the leadership role in these terms. It is true that you may become responsible for meeting many of the emotional and practical needs of a parent with AD in ways that are similar to being a parent to a child. One son noted, "My dad has always been my mentor. It is hard to accept that he now needs me in the same way." Madeleine L'Engle describes this problem in *The Summer of the Great-Grandmother:* "I do not want power over my mother. I am her child; I want to be her child. Instead, I have to be her mother."[6] However, it is a mistake to think in terms of a complete role reversal for one inescapable reason: Your parent is and always will be your parent, and you will always be your parent's child. Also, children normally learn from their parents—but a person with AD will not learn from you or always remember your good intentions. Children also become less dependent over time, whereas the parent with AD will gradually become more dependent, in spite of your best efforts.

Although your parent's thinking and behavior may appear childlike at times, a person with AD is an older adult with a brain disease, not a child. Therefore, you must take into account your parent's unique personality and lifetime of experience. Parents typically fear any form of dependence on their children. Helping a parent with AD to retain a sense of freedom and avoid thinking of him- or herself as a burden is crucial in affirming his or her self-esteem.

How you cope with your parent's disease is likely to be influenced by your past relationship with him or her. If you enjoyed a good relationship, you at least have a solid foundation for growing into the role of leader. It can be extremely difficult to assume this key role but it can be done. Although this process will take time and practice, it will eventually feel more natural. One woman interviewed in the educational video, *From Here to Hope*, remarks,

"It seemed that I was suddenly in the position of being Dad's life-line. That was very awkward for both of us. It still has its awkward moments, but not nearly as many as in the beginning. We know each other a lot better now."[7]

However, even in the best parent-child relationship, it is very easy for you as the son or daughter to slip back into feeling like a frustrated adolescent now and then. The typical adolescent struggle for independence is often played out in conflict with one's parent. If a parent with AD questions your leadership role, the old relationship battles may seem to be erupting all over again. Hurt feelings from your past may be awakened. One daughter described this dilemma:

> My mother still has a knack for ticking me off whenever she tries to correct me or is critical of some decision. I feel like I'm sixteen years old again and that she doesn't trust me to make good choices. I guess the old tapes in my head get replayed in these situations. I forget that I am an accomplished forty-nine-year-old woman dealing with a seventy-seven-year-old woman with Alzheimer's who just happens to be my mother.

Remaining objective in the midst of emotionally charged encounters with your parent often requires the help of others. You may need your spouse, other relatives, friends, or a professional counselor to help you vent your feelings and achieve a mature outlook on your parent's disabling condition.

If you did not have a good relationship with your parent or major issues from the past are still unresolved, you will definitely need help adapting to your changing role. Because of the nature of AD, it is now too late for you to settle any old differences with your parent on a one-to-one basis. Interpersonal conflict cannot continue without disastrous consequences for both of you. You must find other means of working out your problems with your parent, preferably through counseling. Meanwhile, you will need to call on others with whom you can share the leadership role. If you have a loving and supportive spouse, for example, he or she can often assume this role with less difficulty due to the absence of "emotional baggage" that you have in relation to your parent with AD. Without the benefit of such help, you may feel ill equipped to assume your new role. Your desire for relief, even escape, may be strong.

You also cannot ignore that you have other priorities besides assuming leadership on behalf of your parent. Your marriage, children, and other relationships deserve attention too. Your job and other interests may also demand your time and energy. The growing needs of your parent and these other personal responsibilities are bound to compete from time to time with your own needs. You will need to examine your priorities, and perhaps scale back on other commitments in order to make room for the changes in your parent's life.

If you have brothers and sisters, it would be ideal if everyone in the family shared responsibilities equally and fairly on behalf of your parent with AD. In reality, however, one person usually ends up assuming the primary role as leader. If possible, the leader can delegate certain tasks to siblings. For instance, one of you can manage your parent's bills, while another can take care of medical and dental appointments. Good communication is essential to maintain cooperation among all concerned. Old rivalries often emerge if siblings have not gotten along or worked well together in the past. It takes effort to put aside personal differences to serve the interests of the parent with AD.

Siblings who do not live nearby or who have infrequent contact with the parent with AD may not appreciate the extent of the problems associated with the disease, and they may not understand your growing responsibilities. Just as you had to overcome your initial doubts about the seriousness of the symptoms, your siblings may also need time and experience to face up to the facts. Although you may need to be assertive in making your expectations known, patience is also necessary in dealing with them. In their own time and way, your siblings may offer some measure of help. In the meantime, you may be accused of exaggerating the symptoms, promoting your parent's dependence, or seeking undue control over his or her decisions. Lack of experience, denial, and mistrust may motivate this type of thinking on the part of siblings, so you may need to exercise some extra patience.

If you cannot persuade your doubting siblings to change their minds, it is best to call on a physician, nurse, social worker, or another helping professional to convene a family conference and lay out the facts. In this way, your motives are no longer at the center of the discussion. An objective and knowledgeable outsider can educate others about the disease and your parent's need for care in ways that you cannot begin to address. A family conference can be a useful means of bringing all concerned to a common understanding. Moreover, your need for assistance from your brothers and sisters will be justified. If your siblings cannot attend such a conference, arrangements can often be made for them to join the conference via a speakerphone, or you may wish to arrange a separate phone discussion for a later time. You might also consider audiotaping or videotaping the conference. With your parent's permission, you can also arrange for copies of his or her medical record to be sent to siblings unable to attend a family conference.

TELLING OTHERS ABOUT THE DIAGNOSIS

Just as you may have been reluctant to recognize the symptoms of AD or to accept the diagnosis at first, other family members, friends, and neighbors may not understand what is happening to the person with AD. They may lack the direct experience you have of seeing the symptoms unfold or hearing the diagnosis first-hand. They deserve to know the facts if their help is expected, otherwise they may become puzzled and troubled by the symptoms. Or, because of their lack of understanding, they could become frustrated in their attempts to get the person with AD to "act normal," for example, to remember certain things. Still others might be put off by the symptoms and then stop calling or visiting. If kept in the dark about the diagnosis, they are likely to find excuses to distance themselves. On the other hand, those who are informed of the diagnosis usually appreciate the explanation and may feel relieved to have an opportunity to be helpful. Unfortunately, some people do not handle the news well and eventually stop calling or visiting. Overall, however, others usually meet the diagnosis with acceptance and a desire to be helpful if given the chance.

Some people with AD and their relatives may be adamantly opposed to telling anyone of the diagnosis outside of a small circle of close relatives and friends. They may have a fear of being stigmatized and treated differently. One woman with AD noted, "My friends at the country club would drop me like a hot potato if they knew I had this disease." She also expressed worry that their help would make her feel like an "invalid." She added, "What they don't know won't hurt them." Another woman noted, "The last thing I want is sympathy and that's what I always seem to get."

Those who spend little time with the person with AD may not see the degree of symptoms. In addition, people with the disease sometimes have an uncanny ability in the early stages to "rise to the occasion" and hide the symptoms. Physical appearances may be deceiving as well. In many respects, AD is an invisible disease in its early stages, since there are seldom any physical manifestations. The appearance of good health, coupled with social abilities, may give others the idea that nothing is wrong. In *Alzheimer's Disease: Inside Looking Out*, a woman named Barb remarks, "Outwardly I look perfect so usually nobody can tell anything is wrong. They don't notice what's happening with me. To me, succeeding with this disease was seeing how many people I could fool."[8] After explaining some of her "cover-up strategies" for her AD, Christine Boden writes, "After a social chat with you when I might have seemed so incredibly well and mentally focused, I sink back exhausted, wrung out and empty of all showmanship. It may take me a few hours lying down with my eyes closed to recover."[9]

Casual observers may wonder if reports about the person with AD are untrue or exaggerated. They may have little or no knowledge about the early stages of the disease and think of it strictly in the dramatic terms often portrayed in the media. You and others close to the situation may be upset over these wrong impressions and the misunderstanding demonstrated by others. One woman expressed her dismay over the reactions of her husband's extended family to his disease: "His brothers and sisters see him only on major holidays and then they talk about old times together. Of course, they can see that he can reminisce so they assume his memory is fine. They have no idea what is happening with him day to day."

It can be confusing or upsetting for family and friends to be left uninformed about a loved one who has been diagnosed with AD. It can also be difficult for you to maintain a facade and keep the diagnosis a secret. It may be impossible to keep the person with AD out of the way of people and situations that might expose her or his difficulties. And as the disease progresses, it will become more difficult to explain away the symptoms. The husband and son of the woman quoted above, who wanted no one at her country club to know about her diagnosis, admitted growing tired of making excuses for her, though they wished to honor her request. They noted that several friends had expressed concern about her state of mind. She grew less adept at hiding her symptoms as her disease advanced. In addition, her husband felt isolated because he could not discuss their situation with others. Eventually, he was able to reveal her diagnosis to their circle of friends, thus gaining a new source of help and understanding.

As with most issues confronting you in your role as leader, the decision about disclosing the diagnosis must be weighed in light of the needs of the person with AD and the needs of others, including yourself. Protecting privacy and upholding secrecy about the diagnosis eventually proves unrealistic. At some point you will have to break the silence and let others learn the truth. They can then choose for themselves whether to become involved in some way. If there is a long delay in spreading the news, most people figure out the truth anyway.

How and when this news is revealed is also a personal decision. Sometimes it is first done one-on-one with selected relatives and friends. You can also make an announcement by sending a letter to everyone the affected person knows. Such news should begin with the medical facts, especially the current symptoms and needs of the person with AD. There should also be an explanation of how others might be helpful both now and in the future. Finally, the importance of maintaining a caring attitude toward the person should be stressed in disclosing the diagnosis to others. The following sample letter illustrates how the news might be shared with others:

Dear Family and Friends,

I am writing with some news about my dad and a request for your help. Over the past few years there have been gradual changes in his memory and thinking, so we recently took him to a doctor for a medical evaluation. After conducting several tests, the doctor explained to our immediate family, including Dad, that he has symptoms of Alzheimer's disease. We were shocked at first, but Dad seemed unfazed by the diagnosis. We're told that the disease progresses slowly in most cases and that Dad may stay about the same for months, even years. We are hoping that the medication he is now taking will slow down the progression and partially improve his forgetfulness. There is no magic pill for Alzheimer's disease, but researchers are making strides in understanding its causes and developing better treatments.

Dad looks well and feels fine most of the time. Physical problems are not apparent at this stage. He does not seem as quick and talkative as he was in the past, although he still has a good sense of humor. He likes to talk about "old times," but his memory of recent events is getting poor. He enjoys people, but sometimes the fast pace of conversations or the commotion of younger kids bothers him so we try to accommodate him. He still drives a car but no longer ventures outside the local area for fear of getting lost. He enjoys playing golf but needs encouragement to do so, as he feels embarrassed that he forgets his score. He helps with all sorts of tasks but needs reminders along the way. Dad is remarkably "normal" in some ways and yet quite different from his "old self" in other ways.

Dad's disease has been difficult for all of us, especially our mother. Dad is no longer the man he was a few years ago, and this has caused Mom much grief, though she is coping relatively well. She has made many adjustments to his needs, and those of us who live nearby are doing our best to pitch in. The doctor warned us that Dad will need more of our time and energy as his symptoms worsen.

Mom and Dad clearly do not want pity, but they need to be in contact with supportive people. Your visits, outings, phone calls, cards, and letters would let them know that you care about them in this difficult time. Please call or write if you have any questions. I will occasionally update you about Dad's condition and his changing needs. Both Mom and Dad will need emotional support and practical help along the way. I hope that all of us can help them make the best of a difficult situation. Your concern is most appreciated.

Sincerely,

(Your name)

THE REACTIONS OF OTHERS

It is difficult to predict how relatives, friends, neighbors, and others will react to the knowledge that someone close to them has a disabling brain disease. AD can have deep personal meaning for people, both real and symbolic. For some it evokes their fear of death, for others it is one of life's challenges to be confronted with grace and dignity. Just as your relationship with the person with AD is changing, your relationship with others must change too as new priorities arise. Some loyal people will stand by you, others may disappoint you with their seeming insensitivity. Some people will surprise you with their compassion and others will sadly drift away.

You will need to surround yourself with as many people as possible who offer both practical help and emotional support. These relationships need to be appreciated and nurtured. One person may be capable of sharing a wide range of responsibilities, while another might manage an occasional bit of help. It is important for you to know who will really help you, and this requires that you make others aware of your needs. You cannot expect people to know what it is like to be a leader on behalf of someone with AD. Because few have had the kind of firsthand experience you have, they need clear instructions about how to be helpful both now and in the future. Your expectations need to be as explicit as possible.

If some close relationships prove disappointing, you need to evaluate how far you want to go in pursuing them. Some people may stop calling or visiting despite your requests for help. You may find it hard at first to understand their avoidance. It may be even harder to let go of your expectations. Nevertheless, pursuing those who cannot commit themselves can often cause much resentment and bitterness. It is better to focus your energy on more fruitful activities. Don't allow frustrations to dominate your life when you have such pressing priorities at hand. If possible, seek strength through forgiveness.

Some well-meaning people may give unsolicited advice or criticism about "what is best" for you and the person with the disease. Their seeming good intentions may be overshadowed by their unwillingness to listen to what you really need. Encourage them to spend time with the person with AD to fully understand the complexity of the situation. Direct contact with the person with AD could mellow them and enable them to better understand your perspective. For example, you could invite them to spend an afternoon or weekend with the person with AD, and by the end, you may have gained an ally.

AD has a ripple effect on all relationships. This starts at the center with the affected individual and spreads to all that person's circle of family and friends. If you are closest to that center, you will naturally feel the effects of the disease most profoundly. As you gradually take charge of a loved one's life, your own lifestyle will change accordingly. Whether this proves to be a positive or negative experience for you will depend upon decisions you make along the way. This will require self-reflection, perhaps at a much deeper level than ever before in your life. A son reflects on his relationship with his mother with AD:

> What we are going to discover here is as much about ourselves as it is about the one who has Alzheimer's disease. Our relationship with one another is changed now, but it is not yet ended. There is for us an opening, an opportunity that will be our last chance together. It can become a very meaningful new period in which we find new roles and finally come to terms with what our lives until now have meant.[10]

A chronic illness can bring out the best and worst in relationships. Rather than focusing on the negative aspects, this can be a time for healing old tensions and strengthening bonds within your circle of family and friends. The real test of your courage often begins with making tough decisions about practical matters. I will address some key decisions in the next chapter.

CHAPTER 7

Making Practical Decisions

*Even if you are on the right
track, you will get run over if you
just sit there.*

Will Rogers

The changing nature of the relationship between you and the person with AD will often be reflected in the variety of decisions that now need to be made. Several areas of concern, typically involving safety and well-being, come to the fore in the early stages: driving a car, managing medications, maintaining a proper diet, and handling finances. The ability of people with AD who live alone to remain independent becomes questionable and issues related to their personal freedom may come up. There may be a clash between the preferences of the person with AD and your perceptions of his or her needs. You will need to be assertive in dealing with these practical matters, since the person with AD is not likely to initiate lifestyle changes without some direction. If you do not adopt a proactive stance, a crisis is likely to develop. In other words, if you do not act, you could eventually pay a heavy price.

ENSURING SAFETY ON THE ROAD

Perhaps no issue raises as much dispute as the ability of the person with AD to safely drive a motor vehicle. In our culture, driving is more than a means of transportation and staying connected to other people and places. It is also a symbol of personal freedom. Getting a driver's license is considered a rite of passage into adulthood, as is owning your first car. Thus driving a motor vehicle has both practical and emotional implications. But driving is not a personal right, no matter how important it may be to one's lifestyle. It is a privilege regulated in accordance with certain standards of competence, and safe driving is a paramount concern, given the potential for injury and death from crashes.

Unfortunately, the driving ability of a person with AD is often compromised early in the disease.[1] Driving a car safely requires a complex set of abilities, including coordination, orientation, concentration, perception, memory, and processing a lot of information quickly. Impairment of any of these abilities may affect driving skills and lead to traffic violations and accidents. On the other hand, some people with AD retain good driving skills for months, even years, in spite of their symptoms. There are currently no clear medical standards that can be applied to assess whether someone in the early stages of AD is too impaired to drive safely. Consequently, the individual's personal desire to continue driving may conflict with the public's need for safety, with no clear way to resolve the issue.

Just as there is no medical consensus on this issue, there is no standard public policy in the United States in relation to drivers with AD. Most states require frequent testing of older drivers, but this method is not foolproof in identifying unsafe drivers. Most states have also established Medical Review Boards that require drivers to provide notification of a medical condition that potentially compromises driving performance.[2] Although state law may not mention AD explicitly as a condition that poses hazards, the disease potentially fits into this category. Again, however, there is no clear medical or legal consensus to offer guidance. At present, no state except California requires retesting of driving skills if someone has been diagnosed with AD. There is no question that the dangers of driving a car increase with the worsening of symptoms. As a result, the state of California no longer allows drivers in the middle and late stages of the disease, as measured by a common screening test, to renew their driver's license.[3] In most places, though, the decision to restrict or discontinue driving is done informally on a case-by-case basis.

In research studies, a driving simulator and a special road test have been shown to be fairly effective ways of assessing driving fitness among drivers with AD.[4] A two-minute test involving an individual's ability to recognize ten common traffic signs has also been suggested as an easy means to determine the need for further assessment of driving skills.[5] Such tests have not yet been adopted as routine practice. The lack of medical or legal guidance on the issue of driving means that either the person with AD or others knowledgeable about his or her driving skills must make a decision when to restrict driving. While this individualized approach supports the liberty of each driver, it also poses a risk to public safety.

Fortunately, most drivers with AD adjust their driving practices to compensate for declining capabilities. They often reduce or stop driving after dark or in bad weather and avoid rush hour traffic, high-speed roads, and unfamiliar routes. Many voluntarily restrict their driving and eventually give up driving completely. They may fear getting lost, lack confidence in maneuvering a vehicle, forget certain rules of the road, or not pay attention to traffic. Sometimes getting a traffic violation citation or causing an accident shows them that driving has become too hazardous, but usually they are able to recognize their limits and act accordingly.

If a driver with AD is no longer safe on the road and does not readily recognize the risks, others need to point them out. Hearing your concerns about safety may be enough to convince the person to reconsider driving. Honest dialogue and negotiation often yield positive results. A frank yet diplomatic approach is recommended, in which you express your concerns and at the same time support your loved one's self-esteem. Giving up driving may not be a hassle if alternatives are available. Arranging for another

driver or for public transit can ease the transition. If good transportation options do not exist for the person with AD or if their
insight or judgment about safety is impaired, they are less likely to
give up driving voluntarily.

Sometimes people with AD refuse to give up driving, although
their skills are obviously impaired. You may hesitate to intervene,
rationalizing that the benefits of driving outweigh the risks. For
example, a spouse who relies on the person with AD for transportation may see no alternative and deny the growing danger. In
other cases, there may be concern that being told not to drive
would be demeaning to the person with AD. Such personal considerations must be weighed against the more important risks to
personal and public safety. To help you decide where you stand in
this matter, here is a simple question to ask yourself: Am I comfortable letting my children or grandchildren ride in a car driven
by the person who has AD?

If you believe that safety risks of driving do indeed outweigh
the benefits, several solutions may need to be tried before the
problem is resolved. Continued resistance by the person with AD,
who has little or no insight into the dangers their driving presents,
may require you to use increasingly strong measures. In some
extreme situations, even deception may be required. The following methods generally prove effective when you cannot reach a
mutual understanding with an unsafe driver:

- Obtain the physician's cooperation in telling the person
  to stop driving. You will first need to privately share
  your concerns with the physician. If he or she agrees to
  accept an authoritative role, family members and
  friends are relieved of the pressure. Furthermore, a
  physician's involvement emphasizes that the decision is
  based on a medical assessment and not a subjective personal reaction. Since the person with AD may forget
  the physician's directive, it is helpful to have it written
  on a prescription pad or letterhead stationery. A note
  such as "Do *not* drive a car, because of your medical
  condition" may be enough to settle the issue. You can

use it later and direct any "blame" toward the physician. The physician does not have to specify AD as the reason; indicating a problem with coordination or vision may be more acceptable to the person with the disease. Most physicians are willing to assume this burden of responsibility if the dangers of driving are clear.

▶ If the physician questions your observations or the person with AD defies the physician's directive, consider a fallback position. Ask the physician to refer the person with AD to a local driver-evaluation program for a formal evaluation. Such programs are usually operated by hospitals specializing in rehabilitation. An expert, usually an occupational therapist or a psychologist with expertise in this area, will assess the person's driving skills using a variety of vision and cognitive tests as well as a road test. It is best if the road test is videotaped with a camcorder positioned in the backseat of the test car. In this way, the test can be reviewed later to illustrate any driving errors. A driving simulator may serve the same purpose. The expert's report to the physician should include recommendations about continuing, restricting, or stopping driving. Medicare and private insurance seldom provide reimbursement for a driving evaluation since in most cases it is not considered a medical necessity, so the customary cost of about $400 most likely will have to be borne privately. Such a driving evaluation may not be foolproof, but at least it offers a fairly objective way of assessing driving abilities.

▶ Ask the local police department to file a request for the person with AD to be retested by the state's Department of Motor Vehicles. If you explain the circumstances, police departments usually cooperate in the interest of public safety. Keep in mind that retesting does not always reveal problems encountered under normal driving conditions. Notify the company that insures the driver with AD and request that auto insurance be canceled on account of the safety risks posed by the disease. You probably need proper legal authority, such as a Power of Attorney (see Chapter 9), in order to intervene at this level. Without auto insurance, the person with AD may stop driving for fear of being sued and financially ruined in the event of an accident.

▸ If the preceding steps fail, a drastic option is to elicit the physician's help in revoking the driver's license of the person with AD. In most states, physicians have the authority to initiate such action in light of certain medical conditions, including AD, that pose safety risks. The physician can mail or fax a brief explanation of why the license should be revoked to the state's Department of Motor Vehicles. A standardized form is usually available from the state for such purposes. A Medical Review Board or unit within the Department of Motor Vehicles generally handles such matters, and you can usually expect quick action to be taken.

▸ In rare cases, a person with AD may continue driving after his or her driver's license has been revoked and auto insurance canceled. A drastic option at this point is to make the motor vehicle inaccessible or unavailable. A mechanic can install a hidden starter button so that the person with AD cannot figure out how to start the vehicle. Disconnecting certain wires or switches can also disable the vehicle. Finally, getting rid of the vehicle may be the only way of resolving the problem. This may entail selling it or giving it away and explaining that it has been "stolen" and that there isn't enough money to buy another one.

For the most part, neither laws nor medical guidelines are clear about this important issue. Therefore, you are ultimately responsible for making an informed judgment that ensures the driving safety of the person with AD as well as the safety of the public.

MAINTAINING GOOD HEALTH

A few health and safety issues also deserve close attention. These include making certain that the person with AD takes the proper medication and eats well-balanced meals. You need to carefully monitor these activities to prevent potential risks associated with misusing medications and having a poor diet.

Medications

Older people generally take many pills, both prescription drugs and over-the-counter products, including vitamin supplements and herbal medicines. Less than 15 percent of older people take no medications at all.[6] It is estimated that at least 25 percent of older Americans take three prescription drugs daily, but that they are not always taking the right dose or the right medication.[7] Following a physician's directions regarding taking medications requires a good memory. Even if someone with AD is accustomed to taking medications at the same time every day, there is no guarantee that the routine will continue without a hitch. They may take too little or too much simply because of their inability to remember when they took the last dose. Failure to follow the correct regimen can have serious consequences, such as overdose, drug poisoning, even death. Tens of thousands of people are hospitalized every year due to complications from mix-ups with medications. People with AD who live alone are at the greatest risk for these kinds of problems.

There are two ways to absolutely ensure that the person with AD is taking medication properly: Either observe him or her taking the pills, or administer them yourself. There are a few other options, but they are less reliable. One is to count the number of pills remaining in a pill container and then figure out if the correct number has been taken since the last refill. If everything looks good, monitor the situation regularly. If there is a problem, try some of these ideas:

> ▸ Arrange the medications in a weekly pill organizer and count the pills at the end of the day or each week. Keep the remaining medications out of sight.

> Get a wristwatch or clock that beeps at designated times every day to remind the person with AD to take the next dose.

> Look into some of the more sophisticated medication dispensers, available through medical supply stores, that use a timer and beeper to provide reminders. These dispensers are programmed to fit a person's medication schedule and are fairly simple to set up. Also look for computerized devices and other advances in technology that may be suitable for this particular need.

> Keep written instructions in a highly visible location or call the person on the phone, although these reminders may not work if the person with AD cannot complete tasks involving multiple steps.

Nutrition

People in the early stages of AD should have no trouble eating properly if someone is available to help plan and prepare regular meals. However, if the person with AD has been responsible for cooking meals, then some changes can be expected. Although she or he may still be able to prepare regular meals, the variety of foods and recipes usually diminishes over time. Often meals become simpler because of the difficulty of following all the steps necessary for large meals. Meal preparation may also taper off due to the risk of forgetting food left cooking and starting a fire. The person may skip meals or resort to small meals or snacks instead of maintaining a well-balanced diet. The effects of a poor diet may be disastrous for someone on a special diet, for diabetes for example, so it is vital that meals be monitored.

People with AD may also lack the know-how to shop for nutritious foods. They may have difficulty planning meals, organizing shopping lists, and handling money, and therefore they may end up buying less food. They may forget what's in the refrigerator and allow both fresh food and leftovers to become spoiled. Even if a person with AD buys the proper food, you cannot be sure that he or she will prepare or eat nutritious meals. You will need to check such details.

A person with AD may occasionally forget to eat unless reminded to do so. If someone else prepares a meal to be eaten later, the person may not eat it without a reminder. Some people with the disease lose their taste for everything except sweet foods. They may crave candy and other "junk food" that lacks nutritional value. Unwanted weight gain or weight loss, and, more seriously, malnutrition, may result from a poor diet. People with AD also risk becoming dehydrated or constipated if they do not consume sufficient amounts of liquids. Moreover, a poor diet can lead to other medical problems that may exacerbate the symptoms of AD. Here are a few ideas to help you ensure that the person with the disease maintains a healthy diet:

> First of all, you should include the person with AD in decisions regarding his or her welfare whenever possible. You (or another family member or friend) might have to take the chief responsibility for meal planning, food shopping, and perhaps even meal preparation, but the person with AD should be encouraged to participate in these activities as much as possible. Simplifying meals is a good idea, as long as they are nutritious.

> Home-delivered meals or "meals-on-wheels" are available in some cities and towns through private catering companies. One hot meal and one cold meal are typically delivered directly to the person's home. Government programs may subsidize this service for those in financial need. Food preferences are not taken into account unless a physician orders a special diet, and the quality of food may not always be what is desired.

> Another government program called Golden Diners provides an inexpensive or free lunch five days a week at some senior centers, churches, and synagogues. These "nutrition sites" also offer opportunities for socialization. One drawback of this option is the need to arrange transportation to and from the site.

ENSURING FINANCIAL WELL-BEING

Another major concern is managing the income and financial assets of the person with AD. People in the early stages usually give up quite readily the complex tasks associated with handling money. Keeping things organized, paying bills on time, keeping track of investments, and making financial transactions are usually too burdensome for them to handle alone. In fact, difficulty with performing calculations is often among the first signs of the disease. Making tax errors and forgetting to pay bills can have disastrous consequences, while exercising poor judgment in financial dealings can result in assets being drained. Therefore, you or another trusted person needs to step in, either monitoring or taking over financial activities. Exploring how to best help someone with AD manage finances should be done in the early stages instead of waiting for problems to occur later on.

People with AD may be at risk of financial exploitation by family members, friends, brokers, telemarketers, and other salespeople. In fact, financial exploitation is the leading cause of referrals to state agencies that are responsible for investigating allegations of elder abuse and neglect.[8] Sadly, a person with AD may be persuaded to write checks, give out credit card numbers, or transfer property to other people and then forget about such "gifts" or "investments." Con artists use a variety of fraudulent mail and phone schemes with vulnerable people who too often fall prey to promotions like phantom sweepstakes, sham charities, and "get-rich-quick" scams. In light of the enormous risks of involvement with such schemes, you should take steps to protect the income and assets of the person with AD as soon as possible. Some protective measures include the following:

> ▸ Do not hesitate to become involved if the person with AD asks for help with handling finances. Even if not asked, you should volunteer to help out to make sure that bills are paid on time and that assets are managed properly. The affected person needs to formally appoint someone to act on his or her behalf. This does not mean that the person with AD is signing over his or her

income and assets to another person, just the responsibility for financial management. Whether the appointed person will have partial or full responsibility will need to be negotiated. Various legal tools available for this purpose, such as powers of attorney and guardianship, will be explained further in Chapter 9.

▪ If possible, arrange for some or all bills and checks to be sent directly to you (or another trusted person). In this way, bills and income can be easily monitored. Again, cooperation of the person with AD will be needed to make this arrangement.

▪ Be alert to the fact that putting assets into joint ownership or tenancy is a limited safeguard, since the person with AD technically retains access to the assets and has equal control. Moreover, joint ownership of savings accounts, real estate, and other forms of property has tax implications for both parties that must be considered. Eligibility for government benefits may also be negatively affected by adding someone's name to an account, title, or deed.

▪ You can protect pension checks and other sources of income by electronically transferring funds directly into bank accounts. Another option is to arrange for a "representative payee" in which the person with AD formally authorizes someone else's name to be included on these checks. These mechanisms afford limited safeguards and comprehensive measures, such as powers of attorney, are recommended.

▪ Become acquainted with a legal document called "Authorization for Release of Information for Fraud Prevention," recently adopted by the state of California. This document is essentially a waiver of the right to privacy, which allows a bank to notify the bank customer and other named parties when it becomes aware of activity that is not consistent with the customer's usual banking patterns.[9] Since bank employees are often the first to spot suspicious banking activity, this document may soon become a model for other states trying to curb financial exploitation of older persons.

▸ To cut down on the amount of junk mail sent to the person with AD, get the person's name removed from mailing lists. To reduce the quantity of unsolicited mail received from national mailing lists, make a written request to: Mail Preference Service, Direct Marketing Association, P.O. Box 9008, Farmingdale, NY 11735. Be sure to include the person's full name, address, and any variations in the spelling of his or her name. You can also ask the local post office to discontinue delivery of third-class mail.

▸ To cut down on telephone solicitations, send the person's name, address, and telephone number to: Telephone Preference Service, P.O. Box 9014, Farmingdale, NY 11735. Also, you can easily eliminate all computer generated telemarketing calls with products such as the TeleZapper, which costs less than $50. To further reduce both junk mail and telemarketing calls, call the Opt Out Request Line, which covers major credit card bureaus, at (888) 567-8688. Within two or three months, there should be a drop-off in unwanted letters and phone calls.

▸ If you suspect someone is the victim of fraud, contact the local office of the state's attorney and the National Fraud Information Center at (800) 876-7060. Suspected cases of financial exploitation should be reported to the state agency on aging for further investigation; call (800) 677-1116 to get the phone number of your state agency.

ALTERNATIVE LIVING SITUATIONS FOR THE PERSON WITH AD

An estimated 30 percent of people in the later stages of AD live alone, and the number is probably higher for people in the early stages of the disease.[10] Without considerable help from others, living alone under the cloud of AD can often lead to trouble. A person with AD is unfortunately prone to neglect herself or himself and to experience loneliness, fear, confusion, and other health and safety problems unless supportive services are put into place. You will need to assess the situation, identify any unmet needs, and devise a plan of action. Enlisting the help of others with these steps is a good practice. Involving the person with AD in the plan is also desirable but may not always be realistic. However, the goal should be to minimize risks while enabling the highest possible level of independence.

If the person with AD lives alone and receives no regular help, supportive services are strongly encouraged for the sake of safety, companionship, and convenience. Occasional assistance from relatives, neighbors, and friends invariably leaves gaps in the support required. Therefore, hiring someone to assist the person, moving the person into a relative's home, or relocating him or her to an assisted-living facility may be desirable. Although there are many good reasons to consider home-based services or other living arrangements, it is also important to weigh all the advantages and disadvantages for everyone concerned. Clearly, the person with AD will be unable to live alone without increasing levels of help as the disease advances. The time line for implementing changes, however, depends on each person's unique situation.

The preferences of the person with AD living alone should *not* be the paramount consideration in any decisions you make about his or her living situation. Your needs as well as the concerns of others are vital parts of the decision-making process. Those with AD generally prefer familiar people, places, and routines. Therefore, having a helper in the home or moving to a new place may feel threatening. Some people with the disease may feel demeaned or worry that their personal freedom will be taken away by helpers, no matter how well-meaning or helpful they may be. Yet it is possible to introduce help casually in ways that ease the transition and improve the overall quality of the affected person's life. In some cases, the person with AD may gladly receive help with certain tasks.

A great deal of supervision may be needed to ensure that paid and unpaid helpers are properly addressing the person's needs. Moreover, part-time, full-time, or live-in companions are not always reliable, trustworthy, or helpful. In addition, although good helpers may prove invaluable in allowing the person with AD to live at home, remaining at home may not always be the best option for a variety of reasons. I will address this topic in more depth in Chapter 9.

If part-time or live-in help is not feasible, relocation may be necessary. Despite the risks of remaining in one's own home, the decision to relocate has many drawbacks that need careful consideration. The person with AD may see his or her home as a safe haven, while other places may feel foreign and confusing. Finding his or her way around a new home can prove very overwhelming for someone with the disease. Indeed, being uprooted and having to get accustomed to another home may exacerbate impairments in memory and orientation, at least in the short term. Allowing someone to come into the home part-time or moving somewhere else both involve a series of big adjustments. The person with AD who lives alone may resist any type of change at first. Anything new or different may feel threatening, since new memories must be created, a problem at the core of the disease. You—and others—may have to move ahead with the person's best interests in mind and hope that his or her resistance eventually wanes. It helps to limit the affected person's participation in the details of any major change. It is important to note that if you plan and carry out all the tasks necessary to bring about needed changes, you can become exhausted. Therefore, be sure to enlist the help of others in this demanding work.

If you do not live near your loved one with AD, you will need to do many things to ensure that all of her or his needs are met. Caring for someone with AD from afar can be a complex, time-consuming, and expensive endeavor. However, it can be done successfully if the proper people and services are put into place. Professionals known as "geriatric care managers," usually with backgrounds in social work or nursing, may be helpful in assessing needs. Care managers can also be paid to coordinate and monitor services if no one else is able to do so. For further information about care managers, the National Association of Professional Geriatric Care Managers ([520] 881-8008) offers referrals to its members throughout the United States. Because of the great investment of time, energy, and money involved in caring from afar, relocating the person with AD should also be seriously considered.

In the final analysis, you must serve as the judge in all of these important matters regarding the well-being of the person with AD. Input by the person with AD on decisions directly affecting her or his life is clearly important. You may find advice and information offered by others useful in making the necessary decisions, and all the angles should be examined before putting a plan into place. Fortunately, few situations call for an immediate course of action, so you will have time to consider the options. Nevertheless, it is a good idea to have a plan in the works well before the situation becomes critical.

DOING THE RIGHT THING

Although some people with AD gladly accept direction and assistance, others resist any form of help. Most people with AD retain an interest in doing whatever possible to have a say in their own affairs, about things such as driving, medications, nutrition, finances, and their living situation. One woman, Ruth, made clear her desire for autonomy: "I'm not a loaf of bread that you can pick up and put here or there. We will talk about it and I will listen so that I can make an informed decision—my decision."[11] The opinions of the person with AD need to be considered whenever possible. Their remaining abilities should be tapped to the maximum feasible extent. For example, someone who can no longer cook independently may be able to help with meal preparation under the direction of someone else. Someone no longer able to handle paying bills alone may still sign checks while another person handles the other steps.

Unfortunately, people with AD cannot always have the final word about key decisions. The disease may impair their judgment, sometimes resulting in an overestimation of their abilities, so that other people must sometimes decide what is in their best interest. In some cases, it is a frightening prospect to the person with the disease to trust others with so much authority over their life. Likewise, it is an awesome role for you to assume such responsibility for another person's well-being. However, you can be satisfied knowing that you are acting to protect the person with AD from certain risks and to ensure the highest possible quality of life for them. The person with AD may also feel relieved and grateful that someone else has taken charge of matters that have become difficult to handle independently.

It is easy to rationalize that someone you know, who ordinarily acted responsibly in the past, will continue to act responsibly in spite of having AD. Thus, there is a normal tendency for you to overlook the person's difficulties with driving, money management, and other important matters at first. However, there are real dangers in overestimating the abilities of the person with AD. Beverly Bigtree Murphy makes this observation about her hesitation in assuming a leadership role due to her husband's disease:

> I was forced to accept responsibility for Tom's life, something I had fought doing under the premise that I was preserving his dignity. There is no dignity in forcing them to make decisions when they no longer can. It took five years of our marriage before I realized the decisions were no longer his decisions, or our decisions, the decisions were mine. The relief that I felt when I finally accepted the task at hand as mine cannot be put into words.[12]

Weighing the potential risks against the person's autonomy is a tough job. Making the right decision on someone else's behalf can be difficult if the choices seem unclear. Enlisting others' help to objectively assess each decision may help clarify these choices and identify alternatives. A daughter described her decision-making process in relation to her mother with AD:

> I knew there was a chance that she might get lost or get into an accident while driving her car. But I was willing to accept those risks considering that she would be isolated from friends and family if she could no longer drive. Then again, when I later saw that she might be losing her driving skills, I asked her neighbors for their opinions about her driving. With this extra information and some advice from her doctor, it was decided safety was at stake and other transportation arrangements had to be made.

Disagreements may occur between you, others, and the person with the disease about the decisions you make. Advice and support from others are essential for keeping a proper perspective. Knowing how and when to exercise leadership on behalf of the person with AD is a delicate matter. At times, it may be readily apparent that it is appropriate to intervene, especially in dangerous situations. At other times, the choice may not be so clear-cut. In the end, however, it is you, as the person's leader and protector, who must ultimately make the distinction between acceptable and unacceptable risks. Do not be afraid to assert yourself in this important role, and trust in your aim to do what you think is best for your loved one with AD. Learning to communicate effectively with the person who has AD will be useful in guiding your decisions. You will need to develop new skills for talking with and listening to someone whose communication abilities are faltering. In the next chapter, I address this topic.

- - - - - - - - - -
-
-
-

CHAPTER 8

Improving
Communication

*Do whatever your ingenuity and
your heart suggest. There is little
or no hope of any recovery in
memory. But a man does not
consist of memory alone. He has
feelings, will, sensibilities, moral
being... and it is here that you
find ways to touch him. In the
realm of the individual, there
may be much that you can do.*

A. R. Luria (Russian neuropsychologist)

In general terms, communication refers to the sending and receiving of messages. Good communication implies that both parties in an exchange share equal responsibility for sending and receiving messages. For example, if you speak to me, you expect me to listen, and vice versa. Many of the abilities that are required in good communication are diminished by AD. Although speaking and listening may appear to be relatively simple tasks, they rely on complex brain functions that become damaged in the course of the disease. First, an idea must be generated or organized. Second, it must be expressed, verbally or nonverbally. Finally, the idea must be received or comprehended by another person. These few steps require memory, language, perception, judgment, and the ability to process information quickly, yet one or all of these brain functions may be impaired in the early stages of AD. In this chapter, I will first describe a variety of communication problems that arise in the early stages of the disease and then explain ways of addressing these problems.

COMMUNICATION DIFFICULTIES

A great deal of human interaction depends on our ability to remember new information and to share experiences. If learning is no longer possible due to the brain's inability to store new facts, communication becomes a daily challenge. People with AD usually make strenuous efforts to meet this challenge but fall short, no matter how hard they try. Because of the related frustration and embarrassment, they may avoid circumstances that will reveal their communication difficulties. The burden of helping them falls to others who have the capacity to change the ways in which they communicate.

In *Dementia Reconsidered*, psychologist Tom Kitwood uses a sports analogy to describe the role of the leader in communicating with someone who has AD:

> It is like being a rather resourceful tennis coach, keeping a rally going with a novice; whatever shot is attempted, provided it goes over the net, the coach will create something from it, and make a return that can enable the rally to continue. The coach needs attitudes and skills very different from those required to win a game with a player of the same standard; but this kind of play can be creative, demanding and intensely satisfying.[1]

In general, someone in the early stages of AD is usually able to communicate effectively, as long as others provide some help. Table 8.1 (page 140) lists some communication problems that may occur in the early stages of the disease.

Table 8.1: Communication Difficulties Associated with Alzheimer's Disease in the Early Stages

▸ Difficulty finding the right words

▸ Difficulty comprehending abstract language

▸ Difficulty talking on the telephone

▸ Repeating questions or statements

▸ Digressing

▸ Difficulty solving problems

▸ Difficulty filtering out sights and sounds

Difficulty Finding the Right Words

Although they might still be able to form complete sentences and to think logically, many people in the early stages of AD have difficulty finding the right words while in a conversation or remembering the correct name of an object or person. The overall richness of their vocabulary may diminish and they may resort to using stock phrases or words to cover up, using phrases like "It beats me!" or "Can't say as I do." They may also substitute general terms for specific words, saying, "I want to go to the prayer place" when they mean a church, or referring to their "money thing" instead of wallet or purse. Some people in the early stages use words such as *thingamajig* or *whatchamacallit*. They may also substitute related words, such as "coffee" for "tea" or "sugar" for "salt." Their difficulty with naming objects or finding the correct word may lead to long pauses between words and thoughts, which can prove exasperating for the other party in conversation.

Dick Barlow, who has AD, writes of this difficulty: "The main problem is that I start to say something, and suddenly I don't know what I'm saying. I don't know how to say it, and whatever I was going to say is gone. The subject matter, the means of communication, the words I'm about to use next, they disappear. It's nerve-wracking."[2] One woman with AD offers a way in which others can help:

There are times when I cannot find the right word. It simply disappears. If I let my mind go blank it will often come to me. Sometimes I will lose my train of thought altogether. When I'm asked a question, it may take a while to organize my answer. If I am given the chance to collect my thoughts, I can usually have a fairly normal conversation.

In addition, people with AD who acquired a second or third language may become less fluent in these languages. They may gradually revert to their first language, since it is ingrained in their long-term memory. A man noticed this change in his mother: "She emigrated to America from Poland at the age of thirteen. She became fluent in English within a few years and then spoke Polish occasionally. But now she is using Polish words more often to convey her thoughts. Her fluency with English is diminishing."

Difficulty Comprehending Abstract Language

Although most people in the early stages of AD are able to understand simple and concrete words, they are likely to have trouble with abstract language. Figures of speech, slang, proverbs, idioms, sarcasm, innuendoes, jokes, and homonyms may variously be difficult for people with AD to understand. Likewise, using pronouns like "him" or "his" instead of referring to someone by name may be confusing to them. They may find it difficult to keep track of long conversations, especially those filled with details that may be hard to remember.

Above all, people with AD need to be given much more time than the average person to respond to a question because of their difficulty with interpreting the spoken word and formulating an immediate response. Their comprehension may also be hampered by any distracting background noise.

In *My Journey into Alzheimer's Disease*, Robert Davis describes how hard it was for him to keep up with conversations:

In my present condition, just seven months since diagnosis, there are times when I feel normal. At other times I cannot follow what is going on around me; as the conversation whips too fast from person to person before I have processed one comment, the thread has moved to another person or another topic, and I am left isolated from the action—alone in a crowd. If I press myself with greatest concentration to keep up, I feel as though something short-circuits in my brain.[3]

The problem of being outpaced by the seemingly rapid speech of others appears to be a common experience among people with AD. In A *View from Within*, Thaddeus Raushi describes coping with this problem:

Sometimes I just have to step back, get my mind off everything, and relax for a few moments after a conversation. I often find myself taking a deep breath such as the kind that follows an emotional event or tear-filled event. There is a period of recovery.[4]

Difficulty Talking on the Telephone

Related to the difficulty with comprehension are several difficulties with using a telephone. Face-to-face conversations may be successful, but talking on the telephone involves decoding the speech of others without the benefit of visual cues. Christine Boden writes:

It's hard for me sometimes to understand what people are saying to me because I miss the first word or so, and cannot make sense of the rest of the sentence. This is particularly true on the phone, where there are no visual clues or a context to help me try to work out what the topic is."[5] Also, dialing the telephone requires the ability to recall a phone number or to find it in a phone book. Moreover, if a message is taken over the telephone, then it must be remembered or written down.

It is no wonder that most people with AD shy away from communicating by telephone. One young man described his initial misunderstanding of his mother's abrupt manner on the phone:

When I would call her, she would use every excuse to cut short our conversations. I thought that she was irritated with me for some unknown reason. It took me a while to catch on to the fact that she could not tolerate the confusion involved with talking on the phone.

Repeating Questions or Statements

A rather common feature of AD is the tendency for the affected person to repeat the same question or statement many times. The repetitions may take place just minutes apart. The listener may wonder if the person is doing this on purpose to get attention, since it can be hard to imagine that anyone can forget things so quickly. Yet, each time, the person with AD believes she or he is asking it for the first time. Repetitive questions or statements can also be a compulsive way of trying to remember, ease anxiety, or become oriented to one's surroundings. As a result, instead of shying away from the phone, some people with AD resort to calling at all hours of the day or night with the same questions or concerns.

One woman recounted how her mother began to call her repeatedly:

> She was scheduled to see the doctor and would call me a dozen times a day about the appointment. She was so mixed up about the date that every day seemed to her like the appointment day. I lost my temper with her a few times and stopped answering the phone at times too. She would call me late at night with the very same question: "When are you taking me to the doctor's office?" It was hard to imagine that she could be so forgetful within minutes after I had given her the same information.

Obviously, patience and understanding are needed in dealing with an affected person's repetitive questions. Determining if the repetitiveness stems from an unmet need may help. Distracting the person's attention from his or her pressing concern may also be effective.

Digressing

Digressing, getting off track, or talking in circles may also happen to people in the early stages of AD. Their attempts to communicate may sometimes seem like free association to the listener. Their speech may be imprecise, rather wordy, and repetitive. In addition, many people with AD fill conversations with irrelevant details as a way of compensating for their lost vocabulary or poor concentration. One woman with AD described her difficulty this way:

> The first symptom that I noticed had to do with my responses to questions. People would ask me a question and I would give them a quick answer, and invariably it was wrong. I would have to say, "Oh, I'm sorry, I meant this." The second response was always better than the first one. I used to be able to give instantaneous answers but now I can't. It's like my train goes off the track at times.

Difficulty Solving Problems

Everyday life can become a series of problems for people with AD. At one time they were able to perform the simple tasks of life, such as driving and cooking, automatically, almost without thinking. However, since the disease disrupts normal thinking and behavior, customary ways of problem solving become less familiar and confusing. At the same time, others' expectations may not have changed, leading to misunderstanding and conflict.

As high school students, we learned how to solve geometry problems using the Pythagorean theorem ($A^2 + B^2 = C^2$), but most of us have gradually forgotten this formula. Although we could once use this information with relative ease, we can no longer remember it since there is no regular need to use it. Because this formula is no longer part of our problem-solving repertoire, we have simply relegated it to the brain's "trivia bin." For those with AD, the skills for solving problems are like trying to remember that old geometry formula. They experience frustration, particularly if someone else is not on hand to provide detailed reminders or direction.

Difficulty Filtering Out Sights and Sounds

Excessive stimulation of the senses through too many competing sights and sounds, or "sensory overload," may trigger confusion in people with AD, which then further complicates communication. They may cope poorly with too many people, too much noise, too much visual input, or too many activities. They may feel overwhelmed by too much information at the same time. It is as if the brain can no longer filter stimuli adequately. Consequently, it becomes saturated and cannot take in any more information, just as heavy rainfall causes flooding when the earth cannot hold any more water. Quite naturally, someone with AD may withdraw or become upset by situations that they find overstimulating.

The amount of stimulation that people with AD can tolerate may be in sharp contrast with their past ability. It may be difficult for others to realize just how little stimulation it takes for someone with AD to become mentally tired. On the other hand, this does not mean that all stimuli should be radically reduced or eliminated. Little or no stimulation can also breed boredom, anxiety, or depression. Rather, the proper balance of stimulation that can be well tolerated must be found for each individual. The following two personal accounts highlight the complications of sensory overload.

Robert Davis describes one harrowing experience while visiting a theme park at Disney World with his family. His resulting exhaustion led to a sudden worsening of his memory and language that lasted for six days. He comments that he learned to be less adventurous and adds, "Fear and tension fill me before any new event, even a wonderful event. I have to stay close to home and have less mental and emotional stimulation if I am going to have a normal and peaceful life."[6]

Christine Boden also writes about minimizing or preventing sensory overload: "The noisy environment seems to reverberate inside my head, and it just gets too confusing for my brain to sift out any sense from what I hear. The world suddenly becomes remote, distant and disconnected from me. I feel worn out, wrung out, and desperate to lie down with my eyes closed."[7] She later discovers an easy way to avoid overstimulation:

> Waiting in the quiet area of the airport, I am reveling in the newfound joy of earplugs. I sit as if isolated from all around me, with all sounds muted, muffled, distant—feeling like a deep-sea diver—watching planes and trucks on the tarmac, as

restful and hushed as if they were tropical fish. No more struggling to keep up with a busy, multi-tracked, conflicting and confusing world.

It seems clear that some situations may overwhelm people with AD with an assortment of confusing sights and sounds, and they may withdraw from such situations or avoid them altogether. On the other hand, you and others need to anticipate the possibility of sensory overload and take steps to reduce or prevent the risk of overstimulation.

REDEFINING YOUR RELATIONSHIP

There is no single approach or set of rules that will facilitate communication between you and the person with AD. There is no right or wrong way to communicate—only the ways that work for your situation and the ways that do not. In the long run, it is probably more useful for you to consider how to maintain or improve your relationship with the person instead of focusing on specific ways of dealing with the symptoms of AD. In this sense, your attitude may be more important than any single technique. Communication between two people occurs within the context of a relationship. If mutual trust, respect, and acceptance exist between you and the affected person, then there is a good chance that efforts to communicate will be successful in spite of the problems caused by the disease.

Most people with AD have limited insight into the nature and severity of their impairments. Consequently, they may seem indifferent about their day-to-day needs and lack appreciation of the helpful efforts of others. They may have little or no concern about the past or future and may generally focus on matters concerning "the here and now." AD not only impairs their ability to remember but also their ability to plan ahead.

For family and friends, however, the relationship is also experienced in light of the past, with a history of shared experiences and well-established ways of communication. It can be difficult for the loved ones of a person with AD to separate the past from the present and to adapt to the changes imposed by the disease. Your old patterns of behavior and thinking may linger, even if you are aware that you will need to develop new expectations of the changing relationship. Adapting to the needs of the person with AD means redefining the relationship and accepting another person's view of reality. At the heart of understanding the perspective of the person with AD is deep appreciation of the present moment. Family members and friends who gain this appreciation often describe it as a breakthrough in redefining the relationship. Three examples illustrate this kind of insight.

Patti Davis, daughter of former President Reagan, describes her awakening to this reality in her book about her father, *Angels Don't Die*. She was at a dinner meeting one evening with her family:

> We were sitting outside on the patio, and I looked at my father. His eyes met mine, and what I saw there told me it only mattered that we were there together. The past was somewhere behind us. It had no place right then.... There was no past, there was only that one glistening moment, and I thought, This is what it means to live in the present. I hooked onto him right then, like Wendy holding on to Peter Pan—I learned to fly over the past into the bright blue space that was right in front of me.[8]

Filmmaker Deborah Hoffman describes a similar realization in *Complaints of a Dutiful Daughter*, a documentary film about her mother with AD:

> For the longest time I insisted upon truth and reality being important. So she would say it's April when it was really May. And I would say, "Oh no, it's May." And finally it dawned on me, "What does it matter?" First she'll say, "It's May?" and then the next minute she won't remember that it's May anyhow. Secondly, what does it matter if she thinks it's April?[9]

One man was bewildered by his wife's inability to recognize her problems with memory, judgment, and language. She was well educated and highly intelligent and in the past could be counted on to tackle virtually any problem. Her husband tried in vain at first to make her remember things. He often pointed out errors in her logic. She felt hurt and angered by his "bossiness" and his "accusations." Their relationship began to deteriorate. He gradually realized that her hostile reactions were justified, based on her perception of the situation. He adopted a simple philosophy: "From now on I accept that she is always right no matter what she says or does." However, he did caution her that he would not allow her to do anything unsafe. With his insight into her viewpoint, their disagreements eased and their relationship improved. When she did or said something that was a bit "off," he would just "go along in order to get along."

The common theme of the above scenarios concerns the willingness of friends and family to enter into the reality of the person with AD. At first glance it may seem irrational to adopt this way of thinking. Nevertheless, it is the only realistic way of connecting meaningfully with someone with the disease. It takes self-confidence, empathy, and flexibility to do this. Focusing on the present will improve the quality of life for everyone involved; whereas expecting the person with AD to act and think "normally" perpetuates everyone's frustration.

Some general principles of communication are helpful in any person-to-person exchange. However, they are even more important in communicating with someone who has AD. These principles rest on one key element: the willingness to listen carefully to the other person and to respond accordingly. This involves communicating beyond the superficial level of words and connecting at the level of the human spirit. This deeper level of communication values the other person's point of view over the exact meaning and content of that person's words. A "meeting of minds" is the objective—but the responsibility for bringing about this shared meaning falls on you. This form of communication takes skill and practice.

WAYS OF LISTENING TO AND TALKING WITH A PERSON WITH AD

The eleven simple things listed in Table 8.2 (see page 149) can enable you to improve your listening to and talking with someone with AD.

Table 8.2: Principles of Good Communication

1. Getting attention
2. Eliminating background noise
3. Using nonverbal cues
4. Maintaining a calm tone
5. Listening actively
6. Encouraging expression
7. Encouraging comprehension
8. Distracting as needed
9. Providing reminders
10. Helping with problems
11. Accepting silence

Getting Attention

Greeting the person with AD by name or using a gentle touch are good ways of getting his or her attention. Interrupting someone in the middle of a task or a conversation may confuse that person, so it is best to wait until there are no distractions. Visual and hearing impairments are quite common among people over age sixty-five, and these can make it difficult for you to gain their attention and may pose further barriers to good communication. Attending to these sensory deficits will improve the level of the affected person's attention and your overall success in exchanging messages. Getting new or updated eyeglasses or having cataracts removed may improve not just vision but overall communication too. New digital hearing aids are a great improvement over the older types and can clearly improve an affected person's listening and talking skills.

Eliminating Background Noise

To gain someone's complete attention, it is necessary to eliminate or reduce distracting noises such as television, music, radio, or the voices of others. A one-on-one conversation in a quiet setting increases your chances of getting and maintaining the attention of someone with AD. One man noted:

> My wife loved being around our little grandkids until she got this disease. Now she can barely stand them for more than a few minutes if they are wound up. She has to leave the room because of the confusing noise. I've made a point of trying to keep their noise to a minimum.

One woman said this about her husband with AD:

> I learned pretty quickly that he could not hold a conversation if the TV was going on at the same time, so I turned off the sound when we needed to talk. Then I could not figure out why he turned up the TV so loudly when others came into the house. I finally realized that turning up the volume so high was his way of blocking out the sound of other people while he was watching TV.

Using Nonverbal Cues

Providing the person with AD with visual cues, either by means of facial expressions or body language, is an important part of non-verbal communication. Looking directly at the person and smiling will help to gain and keep attention. A gentle touch on the arm or hand provides an immediate connection. Visual cues, props, gestures, and other forms of body language are also helpful in reinforcing verbal messages. Such means of communication may actually be more effective than spoken words.

Maintaining a Calm Tone

A slow and relaxed tone of voice conveys patience, whereas a loud and hurried tone will prove confusing to the person with the disease. Although the person with AD may not grasp the exact meaning of your words, the tone of your voice may speak volumes. For this reason, people with AD will often "mirror" your emotional state. For example, if you sound anxious during a conversation, you may trigger anxiety in the other person. Be aware of your attitudes and feelings, since you may unintentionally communicate them through the tone of your voice and the pace of your words.

Most of us talk quickly and incorporate many ideas into our statements and questions. A person with AD is likely to lose track of rapid speech and become confused. Even a seemingly normal rate of speech can move too quickly for someone with AD to decipher. For example, if you are familiar with another language but not fluent enough to keep pace with a native speaker of that language, then you will appreciate the chance to slow down the conversation. You should apply the same principle when speaking with someone with AD. Slowing the pace of your speech may require a conscious effort. One daughter observed, "I have to really slow down my pace of talking whenever I'm around my mother. Otherwise, I see her getting anxious or drifting off within a matter of seconds." At the same time, you do not want to sound condescending, as if you are talking to a young child.

Listening Actively

The specific wording or content of an affected person's speech may not be as important as the thoughts and feelings he or she is trying to express. Accessing this deeper level of meaning may be your key to understanding what is being said. One son points out: "At times I could not figure out what my father was saying because of his difficulty with finding the right words. But how he expressed himself gave me some clues that helped me connect with him." Taking the time to listen in this way takes great patience but it usually yields many benefits. Judy Bow writes about the importance of good listening in relation to her husband with AD: "It has become too easy to discount his input because it's difficult to understand. Invariably, I have found that listening patiently to his input will provide something I had not thought about in a given situation."[10] Careful listening is an art that requires practice. One man used a handy formula for learning this art in relation to his wife with AD: "I now try to make a conscious effort to listen twice as much as I talk."

Encouraging Expression

As discussed earlier in the chapter, the person with AD may need to "talk around" a topic before finding the right word or phrase. You should help someone who is clearly having this kind of difficulty by supplying the needed language. He or she will appreciate your help. Forcing someone to struggle for words is unfair and unnecessary. At the same time, it is also important to leave extra time for the person to process a thought or feeling before they come up with an appropriate response. It is tempting to speak for someone with AD, instead of merely helping along a halting conversation, but you should avoid interrupting. It is also helpful to keep a conversation on track, since the person with AD may tend to get lost in a flurry of words and thoughts. Finally, correcting mistakes and getting into a contest of wills are counterproductive. The topic should be changed if this happens. Otherwise, the person with AD may feel put down, become frustrated, and hesitate to get into another conversation.

Encouraging Comprehension

When speaking to the person with AD, you need to make sure that what you say is comprehended. You cannot assume that communication is taking place just because the other person is nodding in agreement or giving a superficial response. Therefore, it is useful to structure a conversation by first introducing a topic and gradually filling in the specifics. By going from the general to the specific, the person with AD will be better able to link the context and the details. One son noted: "My father was always a quick study on any subject. It took a while for me to realize that he could no longer keep up with complex explanations. When I caught on and managed to explain something in simpler terms, he was able to understand."

Open-ended questions can be confusing to the person with AD. Questions requiring a simple yes or no answer or a limited number of responses are more likely to be understood. One man described a common scenario:

Whenever we went to a restaurant together, my wife would look at the menu for the longest time. When asked about her food choice, she would defer to me and say, "I'll have what you are having." But if I asked her if she wanted one thing or the other, she could readily give me her own preference. There were far too many choices for her on the menu, so narrowing the options for her was helpful.

Limiting choices regarding food, clothes, or activities to just two or three items enables people with AD to make their personal wishes known and helps them to preserve their status as adults.

Likewise, abstract ideas and long-winded explanations are bound to cause difficulties. Concrete language and short simple sentences are better understood. You should also avoid using analogies, proverbs, idioms, and figures of speech—use simpler terms instead. It takes intellectual depth to reach beyond the literal meaning of sayings such as "A rolling stone gathers no moss" or "People who live in glass houses shouldn't throw stones."

It is also important to remember, when giving directions to someone with AD, that saying something like "Hop in the car," for example, may be taken literally and cause confusion. Try to use specific words as much as possible. For example, instead of saying, "Here it is," try saying, "Here is your hat." It may also be more helpful to refer to another person by name instead of using ambiguous pronouns. Repeating or rephrasing a question or statement may also provide needed clarification. Finally, every effort should be made to avoid asking the most threatening and useless question of all: "Don't you remember?"

Distracting as Needed

When a person with AD asks questions or makes statements repetitively, diverting her or his attention to another topic or activity may be enough to break the cycle. Distraction may also consist of going for a walk or sharing a snack. Asking the person to reminisce about the distant past can also be a pleasurable diversion. Distraction is also a good way of calming the person with AD when he or she becomes angry with you or is frustrated by a difficult task. There is a good chance that she or he will forget about the unpleasant situation in a short time. It's fair game to take advantage of the person's memory problem in such situations!

Providing Reminders

In the early stages of AD, many people with the disease use written reminders to compensate for their faulty memory. Although this strategy can be helpful, they also need to be able to recall the whereabouts of the reminders. One man found success in giving his wife with AD an index card every day on which he wrote down responses to her frequently asked questions. For example, if she asked, "What day is it today?" or "What are we doing today?" he told her to look for the answer on the card kept in her pocket. She eventually got into the habit of looking at these cards without any prompting. Calendars and diaries can be good memory aids and should be encouraged if they have been used regularly in the past. Posting notes in a conspicuous place can also be useful. However, such written reminders should be stopped if they become a source of confusion.

Giving repeated reminders to someone with AD may ease their anxiety over forgetfulness. Yet keep in mind that repeated reminders about emotional situations can actually increase anxiety and provoke repeated questions about the topic. For example, telling someone with AD that minor surgery is scheduled a month from now is likely to cause alarm. Therefore, it is often better to wait until the last moment to give information about an upcoming event. One young woman observed:

> I had to give up preparing my mother for anything. She would constantly ask about some future activity as soon as I would mention it to her. I have learned to wait. I do not tell her about an event until the time I actually need her involvement. Now she is not nearly as repetitive as she was before I figured out this tactic.

Helping with Problems

Rather than posing a loaded question, try offering solutions. For example, in introducing someone, you might say, "Here's your nephew, John, and his wife, Sharon," instead of asking, "Do you remember everyone's name?" Avoid quizzing whenever possible, and instead provide appropriate information.

Although a person's ability to perform familiar tasks remains relatively intact in the early stages of AD, there are times when any task, even a simple one, appears too complex and demanding. For example, there may be as many as a hundred steps involved in writing and sending a letter, and someone with AD may find it impossible to complete all these steps independently. However, breaking tasks into small, concrete steps, giving reminders in the process, and assisting with difficult steps may allow for the entire task to be completed. Again, patience and a willingness to slow down your usual pace of doing things are required to lend this kind of support.

A new or unfamiliar task may pose a real problem-solving challenge to someone with AD. It may be akin to learning a new language in adulthood. One woman explained her futile attempt to simplify her mother's life:

> I noticed that she had not been eating properly. So I bought her a microwave oven so she could cook food without a hassle. She never used it, complaining that she could not figure out the instructions. I never imagined that it would be difficult for her. On second thought, she had never used anything but a stove for cooking in the past.

Encouraging the use of remaining abilities involving "over-learned" or familiar tasks will result in greater opportunities for the person with AD to succeed. For example, someone with AD may still enjoy playing familiar tunes on a piano but will have much difficulty learning a new song.

Accepting Silence

People with AD tend to rely less on words for communication as the disease progresses over time. Nonverbal means of communication take on increasing importance as the capacity and desire to use words diminishes. Someone with AD may no longer initiate conversations but may readily respond to questions from and comments by others. The normal give-and-take of interaction usually changes in such a way that the person with AD settles into a quiet role. It can be a mistake to interpret this silence as a sign of anger or depression. In fact, you may have more of a problem with this silence than the quiet person does! There is not necessarily anything wrong with your relationship, despite the decrease in the quantity and quality of verbal exchanges. And just because the person with AD does not talk as much as he or she did in the past does not mean that thoughts and feelings are absent. Either you can help the person to express those thoughts and feelings or learn to accept the silence.

WHOSE PROBLEM IS IT?

The communication difficulties associated with AD illustrate why others must take an active role in preserving abilities and compensating for the inabilities of people with AD. In a real sense, customary ways of relating to the world have become difficult for them. As a result, communication also becomes a problem. From the perspective of people with AD, we are the ones who are making life difficult.

We must begin by putting aside our preconceived notions about the importance of intellectual abilities and adjust our expectations to the needs of the person with AD. It then becomes possible for us to enter their realm and feel comfortable with the changing relationship. They may not be able to articulate their gratitude for this sensitivity to their needs, but the atmosphere of trust, understanding, and openness fostered by effective communication will make life better for everyone.

Communicating well with someone with AD involves a learning process. It may take months, even years, before you become comfortable with using a new set of communication skills in your relationship. One man noted that he made progress in changing his ways when he began to filter his ideas and words to his wife "through the prism of Alzheimer's." A daughter described her transition to becoming "like an improvisational actor" in regard to her mother's communication difficulties. A period of trial and error can be expected. After all, a major shift in roles is taking place in the relationship, and old communication habits are hard to break.

Reflecting on your successes and failures is critical to your learning process. Ann Davidson shares a powerful insight into coping with her husband's disease based on mistakes she had made:

> I've learned to track that flash of reaction between situation and upset, to discover my intervening thoughts. When Julian does something odd, I sometimes think, "Stupid man!" or "Oh, God, he's getting worse!" or "I'm going crazy." These thoughts flash through my brain, faster than I'm aware of them. But when I stop and tell myself, "The man I love has terrible memory problems" or "He can't help it," I react differently and better feelings emerge. Replacing harsh statements with more helpful ones changes the way I feel. Events alone don't create bad feelings. What we think and tell ourselves causes a large part of our distress. I can't control what Julian says and does; I can control how I react.[11]

Communication difficulties caused by AD may pose the greatest challenge to your relationship with the person with the disease. These difficulties cannot be controlled, but your reactions to them can be. Learning new ways of communicating can help bridge the gap being created by the disease. For further ideas on how to enhance communication, I highly recommend the books listed in the Resources, especially *A Dignified Life: The Best Friends Approach to Alzheimer's Care*.

Communication is also central in helping your loved one with AD plan for the future. The next chapter focuses attention on several steps you will need to initiate in preparation for the near and long-term future.

CHAPTER 9

Helping a Person with AD to Plan for the Future

*Failing to plan is planning
to fail.*

Anonymous

For now, all that is required of you in planning for the future is putting a few things in order. Some of these matters need immediate attention, while others call for careful thought before you act. Table 9.1 summarizes some key planning consider-ations. The last two items on this list are concerned primarily with things you need to know about in the future; these will be dis-cussed further in Chapter 12.

Table 9.1: Key Planning Considerations

- Addressing legal and financial affairs
- Rethinking the living situation
- Choosing a physician and other professionals
- Exploring community resources
- Learning more about the progression of the disease

FINDING THE TIME

Even before you get into the details of planning for the short term, it is reasonable for you to ask, "Where do I find the time to do everything?" Even if you are retired, you probably had other activities that occupied your time and energy before AD entered the picture. If you are employed either full-time or part-time, it may be a real juggling act to balance your job and your personal responsibilities, including those related to the person with AD. It will certainly require a rearranging of your priorities. Little by little, you will need to make room in your life for attending to the details of another person's life. You should not assume that all your leisure activities are dispensable, since they are needed to refresh you and help you maintain a healthy balance in your life. However, you will most likely need to cut down on some of the things you do.

If you are employed but are in a position to retire or scale back your work hours, explore those options. If, on the other hand, work is a good outlet for you, consider other ways of finding time for caring someone with AD. There may be creative alternatives that put some flexibility into your work schedule. Instead of quitting work altogether or being absent regularly, you could explore the benefits of the Family and Medical Leave Act.

The Family and Medical Leave Act is a U.S. law that requires employers with fifty or more employees to grant up to twelve weeks of unpaid leave a year for the care of a parent, spouse, or child with a serious health condition, among other specified reasons. AD fits the definition of a serious health condition covered under the law. The leave can be taken all at once or intermittently. For example, you may choose to reduce your work schedule from forty to thirty hours per week. In this way, you can extend your leave throughout the year. An employer may require you to use any or all accrued paid leave you are entitled to under your customary benefits package as part of the twelve-week allotment. Under the law, an employer must maintain your health insurance benefits and, when the leave is finished, reinstate you at the same or an equivalent level of pay and status. To be eligible for this leave you must have worked at a company for at least twelve months and have put in at least 1,250 hours before the leave. You also must submit a medical certification form regarding the nature of the illness and give up to thirty days' notice whenever possible. One woman took a four-month leave from her job to plan for her mother's move into a retirement community:

> The leave from work gave me time to devote to a thousand details—like arranging medical and dental appointments, choosing the right place with Mom, moving her into her new home and selling her old one. It gave my mother someone to lean on during this difficult transition. I had peace of mind knowing that I could step back into my job. The leave was a godsend.

Time is a precious commodity that should be managed carefully, given the myriad needs of someone with AD. A woman whose mother has AD notes, "I'm no longer responsible for just my own life. I'm now planning for two at all times. I've never had to be so efficient!" One man whose wife has AD explains that he applies his business skills to address this challenge: "I see her disease as a massive project. I line up the resources to help us succeed. I had to orient my schedule to that reality. Priorities now fall into place more easily." This is a good approach to take in attending to the time-consuming demands of the disease.

LEGAL CONSIDERATIONS

One of the first things to consider is having the person with AD formally designate someone to act on her or his behalf with respect to legal and financial decisions. Though adults ordinarily are legally presumed to possess sound decision-making capacity, the person with AD eventually loses this capacity. There is no simple, clear-cut test that can establish when this happens. You can assume, however, that at some point in the course of the disease the person with AD will no longer have the memory, judgment, and problem-solving skills or the mental capacity to properly manage his or her health-care and financial affairs. Mental capacity basically refers to the ability to receive and understand information, evaluate options, and make an informed decision that is consistent with one's personal values. Proper legal and financial planning enables people with AD to choose a trustworthy person to act on their behalf in the future. Certain legal tools called "advance directives" should be used before the person with AD loses capacity. These direct an authorized representative to act on behalf of the person with AD in the future, should it become necessary.

It is essential for the person with AD to be proactive and complete the necessary legal documents as soon as possible. Waiting until later means risking the chance that the person with AD may no longer be capable of designating an agent. The agent's main responsibilities are to represent the stated preferences of the incapacitated person and guard against abuse or neglect with respect to health and financial affairs.

The most useful legal tool available to the person with AD is the Durable Power of Attorney (DPA). Since the DPA ultimately concerns all decisions affecting one's welfare, it is a very powerful legal document. "Durable" indicates that the DPA remains in effect after the incapacity of the person with AD, whenever that occurs as specified in the document. The DPA establishes a legal, private relationship between the person with AD (the "principal") and someone of his or her choosing (an "agent") to serve as a substitute decision-maker. The DPA requires that a second person be named as a "backup" if the first agent is unwilling or unable to carry out their duties. Standard legal forms that lay out the terms of this agreement are readily available, but specific terms vary from state to state. These forms are usually available for purchase at office supply stores, and many local and state agencies on aging distribute them free.

Two types of DPA are available: one for health-care decisions and another for financial affairs. The DPA for Health Care not only identifies an agent for all health-related decisions but also includes directions regarding life-sustaining treatments (for example, whether to use a ventilator or a feeding tube). Since people have varying opinions about using technology to artificially prolong life, the health-care DPA makes known the affected person's specific wishes and directs the agent to carry them out. It is not necessary to have this type of DPA completed by an attorney. However, consultation with an attorney may be useful in clarifying any questions and addressing special needs. The DPA for Health Care requires signatures of the principal and a witness but usually does not require notarization.

By contrast, a living will is a legal document that pertains only to end-of-life decisions and not to all health decisions beyond the point of incapacity. Therefore, it has limited value compared to the DPA for Health Care. In a living will, an assigned agent's authority is limited to making decisions only at the point of a person's terminal illness. Furthermore, some states do not include decisions regarding the use of feeding tubes in their living will laws. The serious drawbacks of a living will can best be addressed by completing the more comprehensive and useful DPA for Health Care.

The DPA for Property gives authority to a designated agent over the management of personal property and finances. This means that the appointed representative is given virtually all control of an individual's income and assets. However, the DPA for Property does not provide exact instructions as to how the agent is to use the assets and income on the person's behalf. Although legal forms are also available for this type of DPA, there may be limitations to the powers granted in standardized forms. For example, there are typically no instructions given about the agent's authority to make financial gifts to others. The DPA for Property is critical to planning for the future care of someone with AD, since it specifies who is to be responsible for using an individual's income and assets to pay for any future costs of care. It is advisable in most cases to consult an attorney in considering the far-reaching implications of this type of DPA. Completion of the DPA for Property requires signatures by the principal and a witness as well as notarization.

A living trust is a legal tool that requires the expertise of an attorney to fully explain its benefits for estate and tax planning purposes. A trust consists of a written agreement and a funding mechanism whereby a person (the "grantor") gives a trustworthy person or a bank (the "trustee") the power to control his or her income and assets according to prescribed conditions. The trust agreement includes specific directions about how, for example, to provide for the care of the person with AD (the "beneficiary") by using funds transferred into a trust account. The living trust also stipulates how funds are to be distributed after death and can be a useful means of avoiding probate. Cotrustees and successor trustees can also be named in living trusts. A fee is involved in setting up and operating a living trust, so although it has many advantages over the DPA for Property, its expense and complexity may be impediments. Wealthy people routinely use trusts for many reasons, including a reduction in estate taxes. However, they can be helpful with handling small estates and limited resources as well. You should seek the advice of an attorney to find out which legal tools best suit your situation.

Regardless of which legal tools you use to plan for incapacity, you will need to make decisions as soon as possible about advance directives. Waiting means risking the possibility that the person with AD will no longer have the capacity to be involved in the pertinent details of planning. If there are doubts about how to begin the planning process, certified financial planners and attorneys who specialize in the growing field of "elder law" can help.

Although it is vitally important to discuss advance directives with the person with AD, it is not advisable to promote the discussion by suggesting that his or her incapacity appears imminent. Scare tactics are not needed if you can communicate that planning of this kind is beneficial for everyone. After all, incapacity may happen to anyone at any time for any number of reasons. Present the idea to the person with AD as a means of choosing his or her own agent and ensuring that personal income and assets are protected. Put the person with AD at ease by explaining the need for planning in simple terms and by focusing on the person's right to exercise his or her autonomy right now. Present the planning as a positive step to protect rights and not as an admission that dependence on others will happen sooner or later. This discussion should take place in a casual atmosphere on a one-on-one basis with the person who has AD, since discussing these kinds of details in a group setting often leads to confusion.

If the person with AD is married, the spouse is not automatically considered the agent. It is best to sit down together and choose who should serve as each partner's agent or trustee in the future. If planning is done jointly, full cooperation by the person with AD is likely. An adult child who approaches this matter-of-factly with his or her parent is also likely to get through the process with a sense of relief for all concerned.

The value of putting these kinds of safeguards into place cannot be overstated. If the person with AD does not complete advance directives through a Durable Power of Attorney or a living trust, others may take advantage of the situation. There may be theft and exploitation by unscrupulous people, including friends and relatives. Someone with AD who lives alone may be especially vulnerable. Your (or anybody else's) attempts to manage the affairs of the affected person, even when done with the best intentions, can be challenged if no legal documents have been executed. Likewise, attempts to prevent financial mismanagement can be questioned if nobody has been given legal authority to act on behalf of the incapacitated person.

If advance directives are not in place before the person with AD becomes incapable of making decisions, the only remaining option is for you or another interested party to petition a probate court for guardianship or conservatorship. Guardianship involves a judge determining that the person with AD is indeed incapacitated, after medical evidence has been furnished, and appointing someone, known as a legal guardian or conservator, to act on behalf of that person. Sometimes a judge will appoint a trust department of a bank to manage a person's income and assets, particularly if there is a dispute among family members regarding who should be in charge of such affairs. Guardianship can be fairly straightforward but can also prove to be a lengthy, divisive, and expensive legal process. It can be avoided if legal and financial planning is completed early in the progression of the disease.

Adult children should be prepared to manage the financial affairs of a parent with AD in case the well parent dies first or becomes incapacitated. It is helpful for the well spouse and the adult children or others to jointly discuss contingencies and to collect facts about all sources of income and assets. Management of income and assets, as well as living trusts, wills, and powers of attorney, need to be reviewed *before* a crisis occurs. Countless problems may ensue without adequate preparation.

Since most Americans with AD are sixty-five or older, they are likely to be receiving Social Security retirement benefits based on their own or their spouse's employment history. However, someone with AD under the age of sixty-five may also qualify for another Social Security program—disability income based on employment history. Such benefits derive from an insurance program paid for by all workers through payroll taxes. To qualify for disability benefits, a person must have worked long enough and recently enough to be insured by Social Security. An application for disability benefits should be filed with the local Social Security Administration office as soon as a diagnosis of AD is medically documented. Benefits generally start with the sixth full month of disability, but back payments can be made for up to twelve months before the month of application. Benefits continue indefinitely, regardless of age, since AD is considered a permanent disability. For people who do not meet the employment history requirements to qualify for disability benefits, another Social Security program called "Supplemental Security Income" provides monthly benefits to those who meet financial-need requirements. Whether the source of income is a government entitlement program, a private pension, a stock dividend, or an annuity fund, someone needs to take charge to make sure that all benefits are being received on time and that they are being managed properly.

Elder-law attorneys and certified financial planners may offer guidance on a variety of tools available for planning for the future. Two professional organizations that provide referrals to their members include the National Academy of Elder Law Attorneys ([520] 881-4005) and the Financial Planning Association ([800] 282-7526). Free information on legal issues can also be obtained from the public-interest law firm known as the National Senior Citizens Law Center ([202] 887-5280). For further information about these organizations, see Internet Resources under the heading "Other Websites of Interest." Other professionals, such as social workers, psychologists, and counselors, may help individuals and families sort out the emotional issues and mediate disputes that often arise when money is at stake.

FINANCING THE COST OF CARE

In considering legal and financial planning, it is important to consider the related issues of costs and insurance. Health-care insurance typically covers the costs of acute illnesses and some preventive services, including hospitalization, outpatient tests, and physicians' fees. However, most costs associated with a chronic condition like AD, which can be staggering, are unfortunately not covered by health insurance. You may need eventually to hire an in-home care worker or use the services of an adult day center. Nursing-home care, which can average almost four thousand dollars a month, may be another option.

If your spouse has AD, you will have certain legal obligations concerning paying for her or his care. And although a legal obligation may not apply if your unmarried partner or parent has AD, you may feel morally or socially responsible for contributing to the cost of care. What are some of your options? Table 9.2 summarizes key areas to consider.

Table 9.2: Financing the Cost of Care

▸ Income and assets
▸ Tax deductions and credits
▸ Medicare and supplemental health insurance
▸ Long-term care insurance
▸ State and federal programs
▸ Medicaid
▸ Reverse mortgages
▸ Viatical settlements

Income and Assets

The bulk of home care and nursing-home care expenses are paid for privately, that is, out of one's own pocket. The income and assets of a person with AD, as well as the joint income and assets of a married couple, may eventually be tapped and perhaps nearly depleted. Expectations about receiving an inheritance should be put aside in favor of the more immediate needs of the person with AD. Every type of income, asset, and expense must be reviewed. If possible, consult a certified financial planner for assistance with the planning process.

Many older individuals and couples who lived through the Great Depression developed a habit of saving or investing their money to prepare for the possibility of hard financial times in the future. They may be reluctant to use their financial resources, fearing that even harder times may lie ahead. One woman noted:

> My husband and I have been saving for a rainy day. It's hard to believe that the rainy day has arrived now that he has Alzheimer's. My son says it's raining cats and dogs, so I might as well get used to paying for new priorities. I did not expect we would have to use our hard-earned money in this way. Who expects this disease? Dying quietly in your sleep without a painful or expensive illness is a fantasy.

Nevertheless, if your spouse has AD, your own future care must be factored into the planning process as well.

Balancing the real and potential needs of one or two people both now and in the future is no easy task, so every aspect of financial worth must be examined. For example, the chief asset of most older people is their home. They may have a fixed income but have substantial equity in their home. Federal law in the United States offers tax exclusion from the sale of a principal residence for people aged fifty-five or older for up to $250,000 for single individuals or $500,000 for married taxpayers filing a joint return. Liquidating this asset may be a good option for some people but not for others.

Tax Deductions and Credits

Taxpayers in the United States can claim itemized deductions for medical, maintenance, and personal care services to the extent that they exceed 7.5 percent of their adjusted gross income.[1]

Deductions also apply to long-term-care expenses. Health-care professionals recommend that you document the need for such services and keep records of all expenses and payments. Services may include those provided at home by paid workers or expenses incurred at an adult day center or a residential care facility. If itemized deductions do not apply, a tax credit for "household and dependent care" may be available if the person with AD resides with you. How tax laws affect you depends on your situation. I recommend that you seek advice from a tax professional to make sure that you get the benefits you deserve. The Internal Revenue Service may also be contacted at (800) 829-3676 for the following free publications regarding tax deductions: Medical and Dental Expenses (Publication 502) and Child and Dependent Care Expenses (Publication 503).

Medicare and Supplemental Health Insurance

Medicare is the federal health insurance program for Americans aged sixty-five and older. People under age sixty-five are also eligible for Medicare after receiving Social Security disability benefits for twenty-four months. Unfortunately, you will not be able to count on Medicare for any help with long-term care, since it was created primarily to offset the costs of acute medical conditions and does not pay for in-home care or nursing-home care except under narrow conditions for a limited time. Medicare and private insurance generally do not cover the costs associated with the care of persons with AD or most other chronic diseases. Likewise, supplemental insurance policies and health plans offered by managed-care organizations do not cover the costs of chronic care. Sadly, attempts to expand Medicare coverage to pay the costs of caring for people with chronic diseases have proven politically and economically impossible. Modest proposals have been introduced in Congress to offer additional tax credits and subsidies to offset the costs of chronic care to individuals and families. Whether these legislative initiatives will be enacted remains to be seen, although there appears to be growing recognition on the political scene that families with loved ones in need of ongoing care deserve financial support.[2]

Long-Term-Care Insurance

Long-term-care insurance is designed to cover the costs of long-term care, but relatively few people can afford these rather expensive policies. Although costly, this type of insurance can prove to be a good investment. The downside is that it cannot be obtained *after* a diagnosis of AD has been made since the probability of using services is quite high. Nevertheless, a well spouse may want to obtain coverage for him- or herself. Since there are pitfalls and advantages to long-term-care insurance, it is a good idea to compare different policies. The monthly magazine *Consumer Reports* periodically rates these policies, and the nonprofit United Seniors Health Cooperative ([800] 637-2604) offers a wide selection of helpful publications on this topic. In general, since insurance does not cover the costs associated with the care of people with AD, most people rely on their income, savings, and other assets to pay for needed services.

State and Federal Programs

In a growing number of states, there are combined state and federal programs that subsidize home-based care. Eligibility standards for these entitlement programs vary from state to state. Generally, by paying for services through designated home care agencies and adult day care centers, they are intended to serve those with low incomes and assets as a means of preventing or postponing the more expensive nursing-home option. For further information about state programs and specific community resources, contact the Eldercare Locator Service at (800) 677-1116, and you will be directed to local agencies.

Medicaid

Middle-income Americans probably face the greatest challenge in financing the cost of caring for someone with AD, since their income and assets must be "spent down" in order to qualify for government entitlement programs. Essentially, the person with AD must become destitute in order to qualify for Medicaid, which pays the majority of costs for nursing-home care in the United

States. However, if the person with AD is married, his or her well spouse has some legal protection against impoverishment. The protected level of personal assets and income for spouses varies from state to state, although the right to keep one's residence is guaranteed. Protecting your assets and income as well as transferring property to others can be complicated, so it is advisable to seek the professional advice of an elder-law attorney. The state agency responsible for administering the Medicaid program, usually the Department of Human Services, should be contacted for information about eligibility requirements and protections against spousal impoverishment.

Reverse Mortgages

Another means of paying for long-term care that has grown in popularity over the past decade involves using your home equity through a "reverse mortgage." This loan plan works much like a standard mortgage, except in reverse. When you purchased your home, you most likely borrowed a large sum of money and then paid it back in monthly installments over a number of years until you owned your home. As a result of your mortgage, you built up equity over the years. A reverse mortgage enables you to convert your home's equity into cash while you retain home ownership.

The reverse mortgage is a loan paid to you in monthly installments, in one lump sum, or on a line-of-credit basis over many years. Your home's value, your age, and the current interest rates determine the total amount of the loan. The older you are, the larger the monthly checks or lump sum, since your life expectancy is shorter. You are not required to pay back the loan advances or interest until the term of the loan is finished. In most reverse mortgages, no repayment is due until you die, sell your home, or permanently move away. If there is any excess amount after the loan is repaid and the home is sold, it goes to your heirs. Two features of this type of loan make it very attractive: The cash you receive is not taxable, and it can be used for any purpose.

Reverse mortgages are considered safe for several reasons. First, you keep the title to your property. Payments are guaranteed by the Federal National Mortgage Association (Fannie Mae), and the loan is insured by the Federal Housing Administration (FHA). Also, before you can apply for a reverse mortgage, you must meet with an independent, third-party counseling service to ensure that this idea is appropriate for you. For information about these counseling services as well as lending institutions, contact the Housing Counseling Clearinghouse at (888) 466-3487 or the National Center for Home Equity Conversion at (612) 953-4474. To obtain a free copy of the reverse mortgage consumer guide, *Home Made Money*, plus other helpful materials, call AARP (the American Association of Retired Persons) at (202) 434-3410.

Viatical Settlements

Another innovative way to pay for long-term care, a "viatical settlement," has become increasingly popular in recent years. The word *viatical* has its root in a Latin word derived from the practice of supplying Roman soldiers with provisions for a long journey. In the same way, a viatical settlement offers the financial resources to care for someone through a long-term or terminal disease. Viatical settlement companies purchase a life insurance policy for an agreed price. Almost any life insurance policy can be sold, including term, whole, universal life, or an employer group policy. In return, the policyholder receives tax-free proceeds, and the funds can be used for any purpose. Generally, individuals must have a life expectancy of five years or less in order to tap into this asset. Therefore, this option may be useful only during the later stages of the disease. For further information about viatical settlement companies, contact the Viatical Association of America at (202) 429-5129.

RETHINKING THE LIVING SITUATION

A question that inevitably arises for those tending to a person with AD is whether to consider moving him or her to another residence in light of the expected decline. The person with AD can conceivably remain in his or her own home indefinitely as long as informal and formal services are put in place as needed. As noted in Chapter 7, if the person with AD lives alone, several options need to be explored: enlisting the help of family and friends, hiring in-home help, moving into a relative's home, or relocating to a facility with supportive services. The option of living independently without some form of help is unrealistic. Furthermore, the level of help must gradually increase over time to correspond with growing impairments caused by the disease.

Many spouses of people with AD often consider relocating to a smaller home or condominium for the sake of simplifying their lifestyle. Other spouses prefer to buy a larger home in anticipation of sharing it with a paid helper in the future. Still others consider moving into facilities that offer independence as well as varying levels of care. Moving closer to family members and friends who may provide assistance may also be a good idea.

When considering the possibility of moving to a facility, you do not need to think strictly in terms of licensed nursing homes, also known as intermediate-care or skilled-care facilities. These medical facilities are generally not designed to meet the needs of people in the early stages of AD. On the other hand, some nursing homes are well suited to care for individuals in later stages of the disease. In the United States, there is a growing trend to create alternatives that afford greater autonomy and offer homier environments than traditional nursing homes. You need to be informed about these different options to choose the most appropriate living situation for your loved one with AD. A summary of these options can be found in Table 9.3.

Table 9.3: Rethinking the Living Situation

- Retirement communities
- Continuing care retirement communities
- Assisted living and other residential care facilities
- Special care units

Retirement Communities

Most retirement communities were built originally with independent, healthy older individuals in mind. These communities have traditionally offered studio or one- or two-bedroom apartments, a common dining area and a meal plan, some housekeeping services, and a range of leisure activities. Fees are paid monthly, and there are no entry fees. It is expected that people living in retirement communities can remain active and independent and will make the transition to a health-care facility only if needed. However, in recent years there has been a gradual shift toward accommodating residents of retirement communities with mild disabilities.

Although many retirement communities have now added a nursing-home wing or a separate health-care facility, many do not have any additional levels of care. Most retirement communities have adapted to the changing needs of their residents by forming relationships with outside agencies that provide additional services, ranging from a bath once a week to daily medication monitoring. These services are typically not included in the monthly fee and must be paid for privately, often on a fee-for-service basis. In other retirement communities, assisted-living programs that allow for certain services to be provided on-site at a fixed monthly fee have also sprouted up.

Continuing-Care Retirement Communities

Continuing-care retirement communities (CCRCs) offer several levels of care in addition to independent living in the retirement section of the facility. The basic premise of CCRCs is that older people in reasonably good health may want to first enjoy independent living in the retirement section but want the security of additional care, should it become necessary, in adjacent sections of the same facility. CCRCs include licensed nursing-home care as an option. These facilities typically require an entrance fee as well as a set monthly fee. The costliest CCRCs guarantee that all types of care will be provided indefinitely. Such an arrangement offers lifetime security for a fixed cost. Other CCRCs offer a less expensive modified plan that provides all the other amenities but limits coverage for the number of days of nursing care in a given year. Still other CCRCs require residents to pay monthly fees based on the necessary level of care. Some CCRCs accept Medicaid reimbursement for nursing-home care when residents deplete their assets, while others rely on private payments or endowments.

The retirement section of CCRCs may be appropriate for people in the early stages of AD, while those in the later stages may need services available in other sections. Married couples in which one spouse has AD may be well served in the retirement section for a long time into the disease, as long as the well spouse can manage day-to-day care. Although the retirement-home section offers minimal services, additional services, such as personal care, can typically be purchased on a fee-for-service basis from an outside agency. Some facilities require that all residents be relatively independent at the time of admission, while others may accept people with different levels of need. Admission requirements and costs vary from place to place. Some CCRCs are non-profit, religiously affiliated facilities, while others are proprietary and privately owned.

Assisted-Living Facilities and Other Residential Care Facilities

Assisted-living facilities (ALFs) and other residential care facilities are usually apartment-style living arrangements intended to serve those needing assistance with daily tasks but who have minimal medical needs. There is no standard definition for assisted living, and many states do not require facilities to be licensed. ALFs typically provide twenty-four-hour security, emergency call systems for each resident's unit, two or three meals a day, housekeeping, laundry, transportation, medication management, recreational activities, and assistance with bathing, dressing, and toileting. The cost and scope of services in ALFs range widely from place to place. Some facilities offer private apartments, while others offer just a private or shared room and bath. ALFs, especially the growing number that cater specifically to the needs of people with AD, are often well suited to people in the early stages.

Assisted living is really an umbrella term for many different types of housing options: board-and-care homes, residential facilities, and supportive housing. In some states, government agencies regulate and help pay for care provided in these facilities, while most states have chosen not to regulate or provide any form of payment. State departments of aging or social services, or public health agencies, can provide information about funding, laws, and policies governing each type of facility in your state.

Special Care Units

Nursing homes are typically geared to people who need twenty-four-hour supervision, who require total assistance with personal care, or who have multiple medical problems. Although many nursing homes have designated areas or units called Special Care Units (SCUs) exclusively for people with AD or related dementias, they are not designed for the more modest needs of individuals in the early stages of AD. SCUs have become commonplace as recognition has grown that residents with AD have needs that are different from those who are cognitively intact. The general aim of SCUs is to provide an environment that enhances individualized care and provides effective staff for tending to the symptoms of the disease. Characteristics of SCUs may include specially selected, trained, and supervised staff; specifically designed activities; family involvement; and a physical design that promotes mobility and enjoyment. SCUs are diverse in nature, and very few states regulate them in any special way. As a result, some SCUs are "specialized" in name only and actually provide very little in the way of special staff or services. As is the case with purchasing any service or product, you need to be a cautious consumer.

The vast array of possible living arrangements can seem confusing at first. If you are considering several care facilities, become a well-informed consumer. Shop around for the best fit in terms of services, costs, and location. Two booklets published by the Alzheimer's Association are quite useful in helping you choose the right facility; they are listed in the Print and Video Resources section at the back of this book. You can also search for options by way of the websites and organizations listed in the Internet Resources.

The pros and cons of home-care options and residential care facilities must be carefully weighed in light of the financial, social, and psychological resources of all concerned parties. The preferences of the person with AD should not be the sole priority. Rather, your needs, as well as the concerns of others, must be included in your decision-making process. In the final analysis, you must serve as the judge in determining if a move is worthwhile. This requires good communication with others who may be affected by the decision, so that their roles are clarified. For example, if a spouse expresses a desire to move because there are relatives in the new locale who will help, then these expectations need to be shared with everyone. If assisted living seems the best option to you, others need to know your rationale if you expect them to participate in ongoing care.

As a rule, relocation should happen sooner rather than later in the disease. People with AD are much more likely to make a positive adjustment to a new environment in the early stage of the disease than they are in later stages. Nevertheless, even for people in the early stage, a temporary worsening in memory, mood, and behavior is likely to occur when they move. Keeping up the daily routine of the person with AD and retaining favorite home furnishings and keepsakes may help to ease the transition. If you or someone else can be available for a short time to assist the person with AD in navigating the new surroundings, the adjustment process will be eased. Within a matter of weeks, the new home usually begins to feel familiar and the unpleasant effects of the move fade away. For further information about residential care options, see the Print and Video Resources, especially the booklet, *Moving a Relative with Memory Loss*.

FINDING THE RIGHT PROFESSIONALS

At every stage of the disease, you will need the expertise and support of competent and compassionate health-care professionals. Every person with AD should have one primary care physician to coordinate care. Physicians of internal medicine or family practice are typically involved in primary care and are often experienced in diagnosing and treating symptoms of AD as well as in addressing other medical problems that may arise. Finding a physician with specialty training and certification in geriatrics is ideal, but the number of board-certified "geriatricians" is relatively small at present. Specialists in neurology and psychiatry may be best suited to diagnosing AD and related brain disorders, as well as assessing and treating problems such as the behavioral changes sometimes associated with the disease. To find a good physician, you can make inquiries through the referral service of hospitals, adult day centers, home-health agencies, and the local chapter of the Alzheimer's Association or Alzheimer Society. If the names of certain physicians are repeatedly suggested by your sources of information, then it is worthwhile to follow up on these leads.

Finding a physician who is experienced with AD and understands its impact on families must be your top priority. However, you may need additional help from different professionals at different stages of the disease. Other health-care professionals, such as nurses, social workers, physical therapists, and occupational therapists, may provide useful services, but a referral from your physician to these professionals may first be required before insurance pays for their time. The primary care physician should be willing to call on these professionals or on physicians in specialty fields for their expertise and experience.

Caring for people with AD is often problematic for physicians. After all, they are trained to treat illnesses and to promote health, but due to the nature of AD, medical intervention is quite limited. At best, physicians can improve the quality of life for those with AD and their families. At worst, they can create additional problems for everyone concerned by ignoring or mistreating symptoms. Many physicians also become frustrated with conditions that do not respond well to medical intervention. To add to the problem, health insurance does not provide ample reimbursement to physicians for the care of people with chronic conditions like AD.

Fortunately, there is a growing number of physicians who are sensitive to the needs of those with AD and their families. First, they recognize that families are the main providers of care and deserve to be involved in all health-care decisions. These physicians realize that their role is limited mainly to providing medical consultation to families and supporting you in your key role in the life of the person with AD. This shared approach to care is not only realistic but quite helpful as well. Second, they make a point of communicating with families by listening to their needs and teaching them about the disease. They take the time to explain various treatment options as well as options not to treat. These sensitive doctors enable families to participate in decisions affecting the care of the person with AD and pay special attention to the opinions of the person most responsible for day-to-day care.

Moreover, these physicians also possess clinical skill in assessing changes in people with AD. At times, the person with AD may have difficulty articulating feelings of discomfort and pain, which are instead often manifested in behavioral changes. Finding and treating the underlying causes of these problems, such as infection, constipation, or adverse reactions to medication, requires a concerted effort. These doctors explain the risks and benefits of medical interventions but emphasize a conservative approach. For example, they will not hospitalize someone with AD except for urgent reasons, and even then will invite families to assist in caring for a hospitalized loved one. Finally, these physicians stress the need for family members to take care of themselves and encourage the use of respite services such as paid helpers at home or adult day services that allow for a temporary break from care tasks. In short, helpful physicians understand that their role is to work with families as partners-in-care.

Good medical care is no longer generally taken for granted by the consumer-oriented public. The rise in medical malpractice suits and complaints against managed-care organizations attest to the public's dissatisfaction with shoddy health-care services. It is vitally important to find a physician in whom you have confidence and who can be trusted over the long haul. You may need to shop around before you find the right physician. Even within the confines of a Health Maintenance Organization (HMO), it should be easy to transfer to another physician if you become dissatisfied with the one you are seeing. These efforts are well worth it, since choosing the right physician will have lasting benefits. Finding other health-care and social-service professionals who can share their knowledge can also be useful from time to time. As noted in Chapter 7, the National Association of Professional Geriatric Care Managers ([520] 881-8008) may be especially helpful in directing you to the right sources for legal and financial help, housing arrangements, and other services, or you can check out the many useful websites listed in the Resources section.

After you achieve the major short-term goals of making legal and financial plans, settling the living situation, and finding the right health-care professionals, your attention can turn to the day-to-day challenges of rearranging your lifestyle in accordance with the needs of the person with AD. Appreciating a sense of "borrowed time" helps to focus priorities during this transition. Making your life as enjoyable as possible may take on new meaning when you consider that time is running out for the person with the disease. Take opportunities to enjoy time together now, since the disease will gradually steal these times away. In describing his outlook in relation to his wife with AD, Everett Jordan eloquently notes, "I know this time together with Betty is not going to last. So I want to make the most of our remaining time together. Whether we have just one tomorrow, a hundred tomorrows or a thousand tomorrows, I want to make each day as meaningful as possible for her."[3]

Keeping your loved one with AD as active as possible can contribute greatly to his or her quality of life. In the next chapter I address ways to engage people with AD in a variety of meaningful activities.

CHAPTER 10

- - - - - - - - -
          -
          -
          -

Keeping a Person with AD Active and Healthy

*I am hungry for the life that is
being taken away from me.... I
hunger for friendship, happiness,
and the touch of a loved hand.
What I ask for is that what is
left of my life shall have some
meaning.*

James Thomas, as quoted in *The Loss of Self*

For people with AD, remaining active is essential to a good quality of life. However, many activities that they formerly carried out with ease may no longer be feasible given the impairments in memory, thinking, and language caused by the disease. Therefore, you will need to help modify activities enjoyed in the past by the affected person, and you will also need to take into account his or her abilities and disabilities when planning new activities. A rule of thumb is to always choose activities that are enjoyable. In this chapter I will suggest several activities ranging from the familiar things that people do every day to more formal programs of activity.

Far too many people with AD suffer from loneliness, helplessness, and boredom. As noted in Chapter 5, the antidotes to these problems include intimacy, community, and meaningful activities. All these remedies include opportunities to *give* or *exchange* affection rather than just *receive* it from others. Accommodating these basic human needs will probably require a number of lifestyle changes. Since the person with AD cannot be expected to carry out these changes, you and others must put the structure and support in place. When you and others participate in physical, social, and recreational activities with the person with AD, you allow him or her to use retained abilities, minimize deficits, preserve self-esteem, and enjoy closeness with others. Shared activities serve as reminders that life is worth living.

You may intuitively know the value of structured activities in your life, but the person with AD may no longer be capable of organizing and following routines without some aid. For example, daily meals provide a certain rhythm to life, but people with AD may become disoriented about time and forget to eat regularly. Planned mealtimes help them to structure their time and provide a sense of daily order. Many people with AD worry about failing at certain tasks and may lose the initiative to try anything, be it routine or new and different, unless encouraged to do so. Fear and embarrassment may isolate them from others, but when provided with appropriate activities, they will feel successful and connected to their surroundings. For example, with such routine activities as setting the table for dinner, you can ask the person with AD to help out, even in a small way. The right kind of activity can also help family members and friends enjoy doing something *with* the person with AD instead of *for* that individual. Such activities enable the person with AD to interact with others and allow you to enlist their help. The key is to select activity settings that keep your loved one as active as possible.

INVOLVING OTHERS

It is important to involve others in planning, initiating, and executing these activities, since you will eventually need help. It is unrealistic and psychologically unhealthy for both you and your loved one with AD for you to be fully responsible for all activities at all times. You may feel that joint activities that are mutually satisfying require little or no effort on your part. However, both you and the person with AD will need some time apart for the sake of personal renewal, so planning separate activities is important. To successfully enlist the help of other family members and friends, a few steps must be taken.

First, it is safe to assume that many people do not know what to say or do in relation to someone with AD. It is natural for others either to pretend that nothing is wrong or to stereotype the person as completely helpless. You will need to honestly address both of these extremes with an explanation of the facts about the disease that dispel myths and answer questions. Your insight and encouragement can help them to adapt to disease-related changes and to be of greater service to the person with AD. They may need information about how to communicate effectively with the affected person, or they may need to learn how the disease has affected the person specifically so that they can help maximize the person's remaining abilities. You can use educational brochures, books, and videos to reinforce your explanations.

Second, keep in mind that other people do not have the kind of contact with the affected person that enables you to understand the demands of the disease. Simply telling them about the disease or getting them to read an educational pamphlet is not enough—give them opportunities to have firsthand experiences with the person who has AD. Encourage them to spend time alone with the affected person, perhaps for a few hours or even a few days. There is no quicker way for you to gain an ally than by letting someone get this direct experience.

Sometimes other people may casually offer to help you or the person with AD. You should take such offers seriously and be prepared with an idea or two in order to engage them as soon as possible. Others often need you to give them ideas about how to be of assistance. It is important to be specific and concrete with your instructions. For example, you may want to see a play at a local theater and feel uncomfortable taking the person with AD with you. Asking someone else to be a companion for the person with AD in your absence is a good way of introducing other people to the helping role. You should be prepared to suggest some activities that can be done while you are away, such as making a snack, watching a favorite movie on videotape, playing cards, or looking through a scrapbook together.

Just as you adapted to the changes brought on by the disease and altered your expectations of the person with AD, so must other family members and friends. In the long haul, loyal family members and friends may prove indispensable in sharing the care. I have heard many experienced family members express regret that they did not call on others for help until they found themselves in dire need. It cannot be said enough: Do not hesitate to ask for help!

People who care for loved ones with AD often say, "You find out who are your true friends in the course of this disease." Sometimes those you expected to help, especially those who live nearby, may be unavailable. They may have other priorities or lack the emotional capacity to spend time with a relative or friend who has AD. You may feel disappointed or resentful when this happens, but if others do not respond to a direct approach, it is best not to press further. Precious time and energy may be wasted on futile efforts and further disappointment. Nevertheless, keep the channels of communication open, since these relatives and friends may eventually come around in their own time and way.

Try to maintain nurturing relationships or develop new contacts. You and the person with AD need people who can provide practical help and moral support. These may include friends, siblings, in-laws, neighbors, children, grandchildren, and even great-grandchildren. If such helpers are not readily available, finding other people who are in similar circumstances may be a good alternative. For example, teaming up with other spouses or adult children responsible for relatives with AD, through support groups or formal activity programs, may be useful.

SELECTING APPROPRIATE ACTIVITIES

Although people with AD in the early stages may have plenty of energy for activities, they often lack the ability to get going or to sequence the steps properly—much like having a car's motor running with the gears stuck in neutral. Without assistance, many people with the disease become confused about how to proceed with even the simplest task. One woman talked about wanting the help of others: "People can help bring me out. With this disease, you can get lost inside yourself." People with AD tend to withdraw from activities such as household tasks, social events, and hobbies if they are not regularly encouraged to continue them. Therefore, your first priority is to select activities that are geared to the individual's needs, abilities, and preferences.

Many people with AD initially resist invitations to participate in activities and need some encouragement. You can set the right tone by narrowing or eliminating the number of available options. For example, it may be preferable to ask, "Would you like to take a walk around the block or take a walk around the park?" instead of asking, "Would you like to take a walk?" The first question offers a specific choice, the second leaves room for an easy refusal. Furthermore, if you make a direct suggestion such as, "Let's go for a walk" or simply insist "We need to take a walk right now," then the person is unlikely to refuse. Once he or she is involved in an activity, any inertia or fear may vanish.

A continual process of adaptation is needed to keep up with the changing needs and abilities of the person with AD. If the person is no longer able to plan, initiate, or complete activities independently, you will need to determine which steps are still possible. For example, a hobby such as painting may require step-by-step direction from you or someone else. Pastimes requiring a great deal of concentration, such as needlepoint or reading, may prove too taxing. As a result, you may want to introduce some alternative activities such as taking a walk or watching a favorite movie. Again, expect a process of trial and error.

When selecting the proper activities for your loved one with AD, keep her or his personal preferences in mind. For example, some people do not like to be served but are quite willing and able to serve others. Some people are content to be passive observers while others insist on being active participants. Although these types of preferences may change in some cases, they generally remain the same for quite some time into the disease. People who have always enjoyed reading books may continue to do so despite their inability to recall what they have read. As the disease progresses, however, their desire for both a variety of and complexity in activities usually diminishes. Simple, familiar, and predictable activities may become more satisfying to people with AD, in contrast to formerly busy lifestyles. Recognizing and adapting to such changing needs and preferences requires your continued flexibility.

You also need to adjust each activity to meet individualized needs, such as whether the person with AD can participate independently or as a passive observer. Occupational therapist Jitka Zgola uses the concept of "activity grading" in determining people's levels of needs and abilities, and the framework she uses

Figure 10.1: Activity Grading

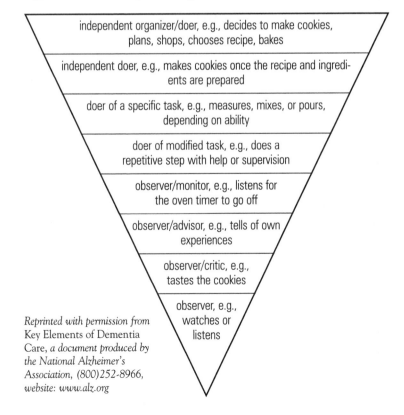

independent organizer/doer, e.g., decides to make cookies, plans, shops, chooses recipe, bakes

independent doer, e.g., makes cookies once the recipe and ingredients are prepared

doer of a specific task, e.g., measures, mixes, or pours, depending on ability

doer of modified task, e.g., does a repetitive step with help or supervision

observer/monitor, e.g., listens for the oven timer to go off

observer/advisor, e.g., tells of own experiences

observer/critic, e.g., tastes the cookies

observer, e.g., watches or listens

Reprinted with permission from Key Elements of Dementia Care, a document produced by the National Alzheimer's Association, (800)252-8966, website: www.alz.org

describes these different levels. In the example on the previous page, Zgola breaks down the steps involved in baking cookies to illustrate how one can participate in this activity at different levels.[1] This concept can be applied to virtually any type of activity.

THE IMPORTANCE OF EVERYDAY ACTIVITIES

When choosing activities that best fit the abilities, limitations, and preferences of the person with AD, it is important to begin with activities that "normalize" her or his life, those activities that are consistent with his or her past and fit into a daily routine. If the person is used to watching sports on television or listening to music, there is no need to break the habit. If taking a walk in the neighborhood is part of the daily routine, then it should continue. Similarly, you can encourage the person with AD to help with things such as cutting up vegetables, vacuuming, or raking leaves. In this sense, almost everything can be considered an activity in which the person with AD can be engaged, at least to some degree.

It is often a good idea to simplify familiar activities. For example, if the person with AD is accustomed to doing the laundry from beginning to end, then just folding the clothes when they're dry may be rewarding enough. As long as people with AD feel they play a part in an activity, it makes no difference whether they participate in every step. Personal satisfaction, the highest possible degree of involvement, and the chance to do something enjoyable together count more than the end result. The process is what matters most of all. One woman whose husband has AD learned this lesson the hard way:

> I used to get upset with Lou for taking so long to get dressed in the morning. I jumped in to help him a couple of times and he snapped at me for treating him like a child. I had to realize that it was in his best interest to let him do it by himself, no matter how long it took. He felt good about it and that, in itself, was pleasing to me.

If the person with AD finds an activity enjoyable, there is no reason why it should not be done over and over again. In fact, repeating the same activity may provide structure, routine, and further opportunities for feeling successful. Many activities that the person considered simple or boring in the past may now seem satisfying. For example, one man discovered that his wife with AD enjoyed taking long drives in their car and was quite unconcerned about a destination. In another case, a woman was surprised to discover that her husband with AD liked cutting out coupons from magazines and newspapers.

Activities that might be perceived as childish or demeaning, such as using crayons and coloring books, should be avoided, although the person with AD must be allowed to define the personal meaning of a particular activity. The affected person may develop new and different interests. For example, to the surprise of everyone, one woman with AD began collecting baseball cards, and her collection became a focus of activity among her circle of family and friends. In another case, a man with AD enjoyed reading storybooks to his young grandchildren, even though he could never remember the contents afterward. Reading together was fun for him and for his grandchildren.

INTELLECTUAL ACTIVITIES

There is some debate about the value of stimulating the person with AD through intellectual activities such as memory exercises, games, and puzzles. As mentioned in Chapter 4, there may be validity to the notion that the brain is like a muscle that strengthens with use. New connections among brain cells may be created through continuing education or other forms of intellectual stimulation. There is no solid evidence that intellectual activities help to improve one's thought processes or slow the progression of the disease after the brain is already impaired due to AD. Furthermore, the person with AD may feel frustrated by her or his inability to perform these activities. The chief aim of such activities should be to enable the person to use their remaining abilities instead of trying to improve their memory. If such activities are still enjoyable for someone with the disease, then they should continue until they are no longer enjoyable. For example, many people with AD enjoy reading books, magazines, and newspapers, though they may recall little or nothing of what they have read. The same might be said for those of us without memory loss, but that does not keep us from reading for the pure sake of enjoyment. If someone with AD enjoys taxing his or her mental abilities, then why not honor those efforts? For example, Christine Boden keeps notes while reading books so that she can review the story line, and she refers to reading as a form of "brain gym"—her notion that mental exercises can keep brain cells "in shape."[2]

At all times, a person with AD should be given opportunities to use his or her remaining abilities to the extent possible without crossing the line to frustration. Pressuring someone with AD to "exercise" the brain through memorizing word lists or concentrating harder on a task does not result in improved daily functioning, as several studies of "memory rehabilitation" and "cognitive intervention" have shown.[3] In fact, efforts intended to have someone with AD "learn" or "remember" may evoke or intensify feelings of inadequacy. Being able to maximize someone's remaining abilities with minimal risk of failure, however, can only help to enhance self-esteem and autonomy. People with AD may still derive enjoyment from games and puzzles if they enjoyed these activities in the past, but simplifying and adapting these activities may be necessary. Board games such as Scrabble and Trivial Pursuit or television game shows such as *Wheel of Fortune* and *Jeopardy* may be suitable and can be enjoyed by adults and children alike. Crossword and jigsaw puzzles can be done with other people or alone. Participating in games such as board games, dice, and blocks with young children may serve two purposes: bringing the generations together and teaching children how to accommodate the needs of the person with AD.

Card games typically require a good grasp of rules as well as a working memory, and therefore may not be a good choice. However, some people with AD retain an uncanny degree of skill in these games and should continue playing them as long as they enjoy them. For example, one woman who had been a bridge player for more than fifty years was able to participate actively in her bridge club long after she was diagnosed with AD. Again, sometimes the activity may need to be modified. When one man with AD no longer wished to play pinochle, he agreed to partner with his wife in playing the game with their friends. Through this simple accommodation, the whole group remained intact.

TRAVELING

People in the early stages of AD may continue to travel and take vacations if precautions are taken to minimize potential problems. In the later stages, they may feel too disoriented and anxious when they are away from home to enjoy travel. Since you may have a window of opportunity for traveling right now, plan to act soon if you or your loved one with the disease has any desire to travel or take a vacation, or you may regret it later.

Generally, the person with AD should not travel alone except under controlled conditions. For instance, flying from one airport to another may be feasible when someone is available to help at the beginning and end of the trip. However, even the best-laid plans can go awry, so each situation should be carefully assessed. It is always best for the person with the disease to have a traveling companion for the sake of safety and enjoyment. People with AD may tire easily in unfamiliar surroundings, so a slower than average pace or regular rest periods may be needed. Travel usually disrupts the daily routine, which can trigger confusion in someone with AD who does fine at home. Maintaining routines as much as possible while traveling may reduce this risk. Having additional traveling companions, to share the responsibilities as well as the fun of travel, may make a trip more enjoyable for everyone.

As long as you closely monitor the whereabouts of the person with AD during a trip, he or she has little chance of getting lost. Just in case, though, the person with the disease should always wear some form of identification. ID bracelets and necklaces inscribed with a toll-free phone number for a computerized registry are available through the "Safe Return Program" of the Alzheimer's Association; check with your local chapter for details. A recent photo of the person should also be kept on hand to aid local law-enforcement agencies in a search.

PARTICIPATING IN SOCIAL EVENTS

The person with AD may also still enjoy social events if proper precautions are taken. Overwhelming sights, sounds, and numbers of people may prove confusing and lead the person to withdraw, so limit the person's exposure to potential sources of confusion. For example, instead of a several-hour event, something shorter may be enough. On special occasions, such as holiday gatherings, weddings, and birthday parties, the person with AD may feel alone in a crowd unless others are willing to engage him or her one-on-one. Several people may share this responsibility, taking turns to make sure that he or she has an enjoyable time. Sensitizing others to the likes and dislikes of the person with AD in advance of these occasions should be part of planning for a specific event.

Even gatherings with a few people may prove too taxing if conditions are unfavorable. For example, the rules of golf may no longer be easy to remember, causing embarrassment to the person with AD. Forgetting the names of others in a small group may also be a source of frustration. A receptive attitude on the part of others, coupled with a willingness to modify group activities to suit the person with AD, will make socialization easier for everyone concerned. Again, this requires that others be made aware of the person's needs and limitations and be given suggestions about minimizing confusion (for example, not asking questions about recent events).

REMINISCING

Although AD inhibits people from creating new memories, memories of the distant past are usually well preserved in the early stages. Therefore, reminiscing may be a truly enjoyable activity for someone with the disease. While hearing the same stories over and over may grow tiresome for the listener, this may be an ideal time for you to gather information about family history. One way to do this is through audiotaped or videotaped interviews. The person with AD can begin by telling his or her life story with some direction from an interviewer. Such taped conversations provide a permanent record that can later be reviewed and appreciated by others. Edited versions of videotapes make beautiful gifts and lasting reminders of a family's history.

Scrapbooks, photographs, and other keepsakes may trigger conversations about personal background and historical events. Some research shows that this may help maintain verbal skills of people with AD.[4] Discussions about the past may also offer valuable insights to younger people and help link generations. Details about one's heritage are often lost with the death of older members of the family who have not told or been asked about their family history. Reminiscing is a valuable way of ensuring that does not happen.

You can also help the person with AD tap into past memories by visiting important places, listening to favorite musical selections, watching old movies, and reviewing photo albums. You might transfer old eight-millimeter films to videotape for easy viewing. You can also assemble a selection of photos and color slides into a personalized videotape accompanied by the music of your choice. Even handling a set of tools or cooking utensils can bring forth old stories. By creatively stimulating all the senses—sight, sound, touch, smell, and taste—you can help evoke countless old memories. For example, one woman with AD spent an hour daily at a local garden recalling her wealth of knowledge about plants, trees, and flowers.

SPIRITUAL AND RELIGIOUS PRACTICES

Traditional religious practices can also involve long-term or distant memory. Many people are members of the same religious organization throughout their lifetime, and numerous aspects of religious practice, such as familiar prayers, rituals, and hymns, may be firmly preserved in the affected person's long-term memory and may be recalled for personal and group worship. Catholics, for example, may remember how to use their rosaries to repeat a series of memorized prayers.

The structured and predictable order of worship used in churches, synagogues, and mosques may be comfortingly familiar to a person with AD who has trouble handling spontaneous situations. Participating in religious activities should be encouraged if they are part of the person's heritage. If possible, the members of the religious congregation, especially the leaders, should be sensitized to the needs of the person with AD. A helpful booklet on this topic, entitled *You Are One of Us: Successful Clergy/Church Connections to Alzheimer's Families*, is listed in the Print and Video Resources.

Music, too, can evoke many old memories, especially in religious settings, and a person with AD may recall lyrics and melodies of songs with little or no prompting. In fact, as the ability to communicate through words diminishes, the power of music to evoke thoughts and feelings should not be underestimated. In his personal account of living with AD, Cary Henderson makes several references to his renewed appreciation for music and the "consoling" nature of symphonic music. Of course, musical tastes vary, and there is no single type of music that is specifically pleasing to people with AD. Knowing about the person's past preferences may be useful in choosing the type of music that may be appealing now, but preferences change. Robert Davis describes his irritation with certain religious music that he had previously enjoyed. One man I know discovered that his wife with AD really liked big-band music, so he put together a collection of her favorites on cassette tapes that she listened to every day. There are a couple of good books on the topic of AD and music that are listed in the Print and Video Resources.

HELPING THE PERSON WITH AD MAINTAIN PHYSICAL HEALTH

Primary ways of helping people with AD to maintain their physical health include ensuring that they get a proper diet and regular exercise. Again, people with AD usually cannot handle these priorities alone and will need your assistance. Regarding diet, there are no restrictions or special foods indicated by AD itself. However, coexisting medical problems such as heart disease or diabetes usually necessitate certain diets, and people with AD often need reminders to eat regular meals. You (or someone else) will need to monitor the person's food to ensure that he or she is eating a balanced diet. Sometimes people with the disease crave sweets like candy and cookies and lose interest in nutritious foods. This craving may be related to changes in their sense of taste caused by the disease. Reducing the availability of sweets and enhancing the taste of regular food may help the situation. Cigarette smoking and alcohol should also be curbed for both health and safety reasons. It is surprising that the person with AD often forgets about using cigarettes and alcohol when these things are no longer available at home.

Exercise is another vital part of maintaining good physical health. Muscle strength, joint flexibility, balance, bone density, and cardiopulmonary outputs are threatened by lack of physical exertion. Regular exercise can help the body maintain, repair, and improve itself. Exercise promotes good sleep patterns as well as emotional well-being. Pioneering studies by Miriam Nelson, Ph.D., and other researchers at Tufts University have demonstrated dramatic benefits of exercise among older people.[5] In one such study, the members of a group of elderly volunteers increased their strength by an average of 175 percent in just eight weeks. On a test of walking speed and balance, their scores increased by an average of 48 percent. Another study showed similar improvements with a simple exercise program using hand and leg weights.

People with AD can carry out a variety of physical activities in the course of a normal day. Walking and jogging are good forms of exercise and require minimal expense and training. If the person with AD can no longer drive, then walking or bicycling to nearby destinations are good alternatives if disorientation is not an issue. Stretching the neck, arms, shoulders, waist, hips, legs, and knees can be done with or without a structured routine. Exercise equipment, such as a stationary bike or treadmill, are also easy to use with proper supervision. It is always wise to check with the person's physician and exercise instructor in case an individualized exercise program is needed. Without even having to leave the house, the person with AD can get exercise by doing daily chores such as housekeeping and yard work.

Structured exercise classes are available through community centers and other recreational programs. Working out at a health club probably requires someone to help negotiate the surroundings. One woman with AD stuck to her routine of participating three times weekly in an exercise program at a local swimming pool, thanks to the cooperation of her swimming group. A man with AD worked out regularly at a gym under the guidance of a personal trainer. Television programs such as *Sit and Be Fit* may enable you and the person with AD to follow a structured routine right at home. Numerous workout videotapes and manuals are also available in modified formats for older people. For example, the University of Michigan developed a low-intensity exercise program for older people with physical limitations called SMILE (So Much Improvement with a Little Exercise).[6] There is also a book called *Get Fit While You Sit* that provides numerous exercises that are appropriate for people with low mobility.[7] Organized games that rely on motor skills, such as bowling, shuffleboard, and croquet, may also be therapeutic. People with AD can enjoy other indoor and outdoor activities like swimming and golf if modifications are made, such as relaxing the scoring rules in a golf game. Experimenting with different physical activities before they become a part of the person's daily life is always a good idea.

SUPPORT GROUPS, VOLUNTEER WORK, AND OTHER ACTIVITY PROGRAMS

Support groups for people in the early stages of AD are just beginning to take hold, mostly in major urban areas. In addition to support groups, volunteer work groups and recreational groups have also recently sprung up. These groups are typically led by professionals and offer a supportive atmosphere to achieve several goals. It is useful to take advantage of such worthwhile groups in one's local area or else encourage their formation within sympathetic organizations.

In support groups, usually eight to twelve people with AD meet to discuss common concerns and enjoy mutual support. These group meetings are useful for gaining knowledge about the disease and exchanging coping strategies. Most support groups meet weekly for a period of eight to ten weeks, but some meet monthly on an ongoing basis. While the people with AD are meeting, their family members and friends usually participate in professionally led groups in an adjacent room to discuss their own agendas. Both groups then usually come together for a time of socialization. Members of these support groups tend to bond quickly and derive much satisfaction from their participation, and some choose to see one another on a social basis too. For example, at the House of Welcome in Northbrook, Illinois, a weekly support group for people with AD and their families was expanded to include a monthly "Supper Club" for couples that has spawned informal group outings. Such friendships are natural in light of the common interests and needs. Problems like forgetting names and losing track of conversations trigger no embarrassment in a peer group. So far, there has been little research about the therapeutic value of these groups for people with AD. However, anecdotal reports clearly illustrate how valuable they can be for participants in reducing isolation, enhancing self-esteem, and coping with memory loss. Members of a group in Prince George, British Columbia, offered the following comments about the benefits of their participation:

> I am very thankful the group was suggested by my doctor. To meet these people experienced with this condition has been so supportive and so much fun. When you're diagnosed, you feel so alone—and then you come here and it feels like a family.

> You don't have to be on guard here, just be as we are. We exchange ideas and laugh.

> When I was first diagnosed, it was quite a shock. But then I came and met these interesting people. It means a lot to know you are not alone.

As noted, family members and friends are encouraged to take part in groups that meet in parallel fashion to the groups of people with early-stage AD. Such groups not only offer useful information about AD and coping skills, but also decrease friends' and family members' own feelings of social isolation. Moreover, family members and friends can witness firsthand the benefits of having a loved one take part in a separate support group. One woman writes about her husband's positive response to participation in a support group: "He used to hide his problems and now he is much more open in letting others know what he needs. I think the group gave him the confidence that having Alzheimer's disease is no cause for shame."

A small but growing number of activity-focused groups for persons in the early stages of AD have also been established in recent years. These groups are usually sponsored by local chapters of the Alzheimer's Association or Alzheimer Society, assisted living facilities, or adult day centers. Although members are encouraged to talk about their thoughts and feelings under the direction of a professional, their contact mainly revolves around specific tasks or events. For example, a group may take on a community gardening project, sort canned goods at a local food bank, or stuff envelopes for mailings. These volunteer activities can help to instill pride and self-worth in people with AD. Like any enjoyable activity, however, the goal is not to produce concrete results as much as it is to enable group members to enjoy working with others. At the Alzheimer's Family Care Center in Chicago, Illinois, members of an early-stage group have promoted literacy by reading to schoolchildren and have worked side-by-side at a sheltered workshop for young adults with chronic psychiatric illnesses. At the intergenerational St. Ann Adult Day Care in Milwaukee, Wisconsin, daily activities with children offer immeasurable joy, especially to many older women with AD who spent their younger years caring for their own children. At Alzheimer's Services of the East Bay in Berkeley, California, partnerships are established between individuals with AD and trained volunteers who undertake community service work together.

A recreational group may be formed separately or in combination with other types of groups. The primary goal of recreational groups is to have fun, but other benefits usually accrue as well. These groups are directed by a professional who provides structure and adapts activities to the needs of people in the early stages of AD. A structured program of indoor and outdoor activities may be planned, but members are usually quick to contribute their own ideas.

Numerous organizations have begun early-stage activity programs in recent years and each program seems to have its own unique style and agenda. On-site activities, such as intellectual games, physical exercise, discussions about music, art, and history, as well as field trips, restaurant lunches, and picnics, are common activities. The CARE Club in Granada Hills, California, offers a daily program of social and recreational activities for people in the early stages of AD. Similarly, The Silver Club meets twice weekly at the Turner Senior Resource Center in Ann Arbor, Michigan. The Council for Jewish Elderly in Chicago sponsors a weekly "Culture Bus" in which people in the early stages of AD take part in guided tours of cultural attractions and have lunch together. The weekly DRC Club and The Company in Walnut Creek, California, are separate activity groups for men and women that also involve guided tours of museums, gardens, zoos, and factories. In addition to community-based programs, a growing number of assisted living facilities are offering activity programs specifically suited to their residents with early-stage AD. For instance, Mather Gardens in Evanston, Illinois, has a daily "Gardens Club" for fifteen to twenty of its residents.

Though these types of groups are not for everyone, they can provide a wonderful outlet for some people with AD. People with AD often need prompting to try out these groups, but are usually quick to adapt to such enjoyable and meaningful gatherings. Likewise, family members and friends are usually grateful for the knowledge gained and support received in early-stage support groups.

BEING AROUND PETS AND PLANTS

In a critique of residential care facilities in the United States, William Thomas, M.D., notes that implementing an activity program is inadequate unless it occurs within a "human habitat" that makes pets, plants, and children the axis around which daily life turns.[8] In promoting a philosophy called the "Eden Alternative," he sees daily interaction with dogs, cats, birds, living plants, and young children as a means of achieving the goal of "a life worth living." The potential benefits of this approach may be worth considering.

Most people have owned pets at some point in their life. Caring for animals can be a big responsibility as well as a source of enjoyment. People with AD may be quite capable of sharing the work of caring for pets and derive a sense of purpose from this responsibility. They may be delighted to have a relationship with a creature that offers unconditional love. One woman with AD noted, "I had so many responsibilities being taken away from me that getting a dog proved to be the one thing that I could still handle well. And my dog expects nothing out of me!" A man with AD reported that his dog provided a good reason to exercise: "I have a dog that needs to be run every day. So we run about two miles together. The dog more or less drags me, but it's still fun. I have a regular route and see neighbors along the way."

As pet owners know, animals like dogs require training and upkeep, and there may be little time or energy available for this effort. Allergic reactions to pets may be another problem. Some living situations prohibit the presence of certain pets. Although such drawbacks cannot be eliminated, they can be minimized. For example, dogs that have already been trained may be available through the local Humane Society. A puppy can be trained with the help of an obedience school. Such initial efforts may have long-lasting benefits. Animals such as cats and birds require little or no training and are easier to maintain than dogs. However, interaction with these pets may be somewhat limited.

Growing houseplants or gardening is a relatively easy way of connecting with nature and involves a number of activities that can be done together or on a solo basis. Gardening also requires effort, but the size and scope of indoor and outdoor gardening can be scaled to meet the desired effect. One man who cares for his wife with AD reports that they happily spend several hours daily tending their large garden: "We have always enjoyed this hobby, so I figured we should keep it up as long as possible. We don't get as much done now as we did in the past but it keeps us both busy." Outdoor tasks such as planting, fertilizing, watering, transplanting, and harvesting fruits and vegetables can be a year-round activity in some locales. Indoor gardening, ranging from maintaining a variety of plants to a full-blown greenhouse, can also be a focal point of daily activity.

GETTING CHILDREN INVOLVED

Our fast-paced, mobile society has created a separation of generations as at no other time in human history. Older people, middle-aged people, young adults, teenagers, and youngsters seldom interact except on special occasions. Different generations within families may live great distances from one another. Creating traditions and building loyalty among family members are becoming increasingly difficult under these conditions. For those families that make a concerted effort to stay together, both physically and psychologically, the challenges of AD can be shared among many members. Even the youngest family member can be affected by a loved one's disease, for better or worse. The interaction between young children and a great-grandparent, grandparent—or even a parent—who has AD can be rewarding or distressing depending on the overall tone set by others in the family.

Teenagers and younger children can have many positive effects on people with AD. Children can be quite accepting and caring in ways that adults find difficult. They can have a calming influence on those with AD, trigger fond memories, and elicit nurturing instincts. Children are often good at engaging older people in ways that are mutually beneficial and enjoyable, sharing simple pleasures like taking a walk, tossing a ball, drawing a picture, putting together a puzzle, reading a book, dancing, singing, watching a video, or doing household chores. Local sporting events are entertainment opportunities that might also be suitable and can be watched together either in-person or on television.

Generally, young children mirror the way in which their parents react to someone with AD. If a parent is irritable and impatient, a child will reflect these reactions. If a parent copes well and takes the time to explain the disease to a young child, then a good adjustment by the child can be expected too. Relationships can become complicated when the person with the disease, typically a grandparent, lives in the household with a young child. The child may be at risk of receiving less attention as the focus of family life switches to the person with the disease. A child may act out dissatisfaction with the living arrangement by withdrawing from the family, doing poorly in school or with peers, or getting upset with the person with AD.

In such situations, steps need to be taken to ensure that teenagers and young children have opportunities for time, attention, and discussion with their parents. Otherwise, they may feel overwhelmed by the demands on them and the rest of the family. Their parents can reassure them that they have an important place in the family. Teenagers and even younger children can learn to share effectively in the care of people with AD. Children may respond well to their roles as helpers to an older loved one who is in need. They may provide great enjoyment to the person with AD and learn valuable lessons about caring for others in the process. For educational materials especially intended for teens and younger children, see the list of selected books and videos in the Resources.

Providing meaningful activities to someone with the disease requires time, energy, and creativity. It is an ongoing challenge, and one person cannot successfully meet this challenge indefinitely. It is essential to involve others as soon as possible so that they may share in the important responsibility of enhancing the quality of life for the person with AD. At the same time, you must also learn to care for yourself. Since you are so vital to the well-being of the person with AD, a commitment to nurturing yourself will ultimately benefit everyone involved. This topic is the focus of Part III.

PART III

Caring
for
Yourself

. . . .
.
.
.

CHAPTER 11

Self-Renewal for Family and Friends

*The apostles returned to Jesus
and reported to him all that they
had done. He said to them,
"Come by yourselves to an out-of-
the-way place and rest."*

The Gospel According to Mark

So far, this book has focused for the most part on under-standing and meeting the needs of a person with AD. How-ever, the importance of maintaining your own well-being cannot be overstated. Caring for someone with AD can make great demands on your time and energy. You may feel as if your life is being turned upside down because of your changing roles and responsibilities, and you may feel tested in body, mind, and spirit. If proper steps are not taken to remain healthy on these intercon-nected levels, a host of problems may ensue.

Numerous studies attest to the potential for physical and mental exhaustion among those caring for people with AD.[1] One survey commissioned by the Alzheimer's Association indicated that family members primarily responsible for loved ones with AD spend an average of one hundred hours a week providing supervision or some measure of care if they live with the person with the disease.[2] This basically amounts to the majority of waking hours every day being spent making sure that a loved one with AD is safe and healthy. Moreover, 75 percent of these family members report feeling depressed occasionally, and 45 percent report not getting enough sleep. If family members work outside the home in either a full-time or part-time job, they spend an average of forty hours weekly providing supervision or care. Clearly, relatives and friends directly involved in caring for loved ones with AD pay a high price for their commitment. Nevertheless, burnout can be avoided. In this chapter, I will address the need for "self-care" and ways to keep yourself fit.

If you are the one primarily responsible for a loved one with AD, it is essential that you take care of yourself while caring for him or her—for both your sakes. Since your life and the life of the person with AD are intertwined, your physical, emotional, and spiritual well-being directly affects her or him. Renewing your personal energy on a regular basis will enable you to meet your goal of providing good care. Conversely, the person with AD will suffer if you are in poor shape. Keep in mind the following analogy. Prior to an airplane's departure, flight attendants instruct passengers how to use an oxygen mask in the event of an emergency. Passengers are told to put on their own mask first before helping others around them or else they might not be capable of helping others. Likewise, your personal needs are just as important as the needs of the person with AD. Fern Brown comments on the need to continue enjoying life within the parameters of her husband's disease: "The biggest misunderstanding about this disease is that as soon as you're diagnosed, you're dead. People don't realize that there is life beyond the diagnosis, and that's what I'm trying to prove. Leonard can still have a good life and so can I."[3]

There are many things you can do to maintain your well-being. You will gradually discover what works best for you. Others may offer friendly advice but you must ultimately choose what is best for you in developing a regular plan of self-care.

LISTENING TO YOUR BODY AND MIND

The body-mind connection is a two-way street. That is, you can improve your physical well-being by maintaining a positive outlook, but you can also improve your outlook by tending to your physical well-being. If you are feeling down, it is more important than ever to eat well, exercise regularly, enjoy recreational or social activities, and get plenty of rest. Routine medical and dental checkups should also be maintained. It is all too easy to overlook these basic matters as your focus shifts to the needs of the person with AD.

Proper nutrition is essential to maintaining your physical well-being, and so eating regular and balanced meals should be part of your daily routine. The Food Guide Pyramid (reproduced below) is an outline of what to eat each day based on the dietary recommendations set by the U.S. Department of Agriculture.[4] It is not a rigid prescription but a general guide that allows you to choose a healthy diet that is right for you. The Pyramid calls for eating a variety of foods to get the nutrients you need on a daily basis and,

Figure 11.1: The Food Guide Pyramid: A Guide to Daily Food Choices

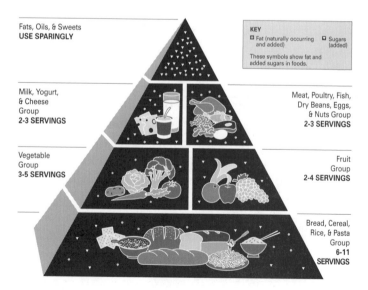

Source: U.S. Department of Agriculture / U.S. Department of Health and Human Services

at the same time, the right amount of calories to maintain a good weight. The Pyramid divides food into six basic groups. At the top are foods that you should eat sparingly. The recommended number of servings increases as the pyramid gets wider toward the bottom. The higher levels of the pyramid simply mean that you should eat less of these foods each day. Robert Russell, Ph.D., of the U.S. Department of Agriculture's Human Nutrition Research Center, proposes lowering the recommended number of servings for people aged 70 and older but stresses the need for "nutrient-dense food choices."[5]

A good daily diet generally consists of eating healthy foods from these basic food groups:

1. Fats, oils, and sweets (Use sparingly, especially if you are trying to lose weight.)

2. Beans, nuts, fish, poultry, eggs, and meat (two to three servings a day)

3. Milk, yogurt, and cheese (two to three servings a day)

4. Vegetables (three to five servings a day)

5. Fruits (two to four servings a day)

6. Bread, cereal, pasta, rice, and grains (six or more servings a day)

When choosing foods for a healthy diet, keep in mind the fat and added sugars in your choices from all of the food groups. For example, there are added sugars and fat in cheese and ice cream. Planning, purchasing, and preparing healthy foods should be a central focus of your daily life.

It is also vital that you incorporate exercise into your daily routine. Activities such as housekeeping and gardening are usually not strenuous enough to burn enough calories or to get your heart and lungs really working. Join a health club, or try out yoga, weight training, jogging, or aerobics. If these don't appeal to you, then take a brisk walk for a mile or ride a stationary bike every day. You can play golf or swim alone or with others. But whether you choose a solo or group activity, the key is to be regularly physically active. One man whose wife has AD notes, "I try to do something for about an hour every day—mostly walking and bicycling but some canoeing and cross-country skiing when weather permits. I probably do more than necessary, but I feel pretty good. Doing something can start a cycle of feeling better, doing more, and feeling even better."[6] One woman whose husband has the disease reports, "I attend a fitness center four mornings a week. The strenuous workouts help to relieve tension and keep me in good shape. It's a wonderful outlet for me."[7] Of course, exercising regularly means taking a break from your other responsibilities. Therefore, you may need to ask others to attend to the person with AD in your absence.

To keep a balanced perspective, it is also important for you to engage in recreational or social activities. Whether you do this with or without the person with AD is a judgment call. Although spending quality time together benefits your relationship, some time away from the person with AD now and then is essential. Attending a sporting event, a play, a movie, a concert, or a party can recharge your batteries. These activities also serve to remind you that caring for someone with AD is not the only focus of your life and that you deserve to enjoy yourself. And, as stated above, doing something for yourself will also have direct benefits for your loved one with AD.

It is also important to maintain proper sleeping habits. Although the amount of sleep needed varies from person to person, try to establish a routine that is restful for you. Problems with falling asleep or staying asleep are fairly common and may have many causes, such as anxiety, depression, and intake of alcohol and caffeine. Sleep deprivation can have consequences beyond feeling tired and irritable, such as triggering illnesses. It is a good idea to seek professional help if you cannot find a simple solution to sleep problems.

In spite of your good habits, you may find yourself feeling depressed, angry, or anxious. These feelings may actually get in the way of your eating, exercising, and sleeping properly. Temporarily feeling blue is one matter, but chronically feeling tired, worried, or sad may be signs of major depression. If you think this may be the case, you should seek professional help, beginning with your physician. Oftentimes the grief associated with caring for a loved one with AD is at the root of depression. Regardless of its underlying causes, depression should be taken seriously and treated promptly. Fortunately, many good treatments for depression are now available, as discussed in Chapter 2.

THE IMPORTANCE OF GRIEF

Over thirty years ago, Elisabeth Kübler-Ross, M.D., described the psychological process of grief experienced by her terminally ill cancer patients in her landmark book, *On Death and Dying*.[8] Her insights led to a better understanding of grief as a normal human reaction to loss and of the stages involved in coming to terms with loss. You and others caring for the person with AD also face a long series of changes and losses as the disease unfolds. Family members and friends often refer to "the long good-bye" in describing their experience of slowly losing a loved one to the disease. Feelings of sadness, disappointment, frustration, and confusion over the losses and changes related to AD are quite natural and may be intense from time to time. Ignoring your normal expressions of grief may lead to your becoming stuck in depression, anger, or isolation from others. Physical signs of grief such as weakness, insomnia, and loss of appetite may also take their toll. Paying attention to your own grief can help you to cope more effectively and adjust to the losses you experience.

According to Dr. Kübler-Ross, grief generally progresses through the following stages:

Denial. Denial is a natural defense mechanism that helps us to avoid or lessen the impact of a painful event. It is a way of holding onto the past and avoiding current reality. Statements like "I can't believe this is happening" or "This is not such a big deal" or "It can't be Alzheimer's" are all forms of denial. Although denial is a healthy and normal means of coping for a short while, prolonged denial can block the need for action. If the needs of the person with AD are minimized or overlooked, then denial may be harmful. One daughter advises, "The biggest thing is getting over the denial hump. As long as you think that Alzheimer's cannot be identified until autopsy, there is that grain of doubt. You have got to trust the doctor about the diagnosis and then just go ahead and deal with it."

Anger and Depression.   Feelings of anger and depression often become noticeable as denial gives way to the reality of loss. Anger may be directed toward God, health-care professionals, family members, friends, and the person with the disease, or even toward yourself. Anger may also turn inward, resulting in social isolation, sadness, and depression. Because you are unable to control your circumstances, anger and depression are legitimate responses to your situation. However, there is a danger in allowing these feelings to dominate your thoughts and actions indefinitely. One husband points out:

> It is necessary to feel the pain for about three or four months, but after that you have to deal with the fact that you are the sole support for this individual. You have to allow yourself to feel the pain at first and then go on to deal with the practical issues of everyday life.

Letting go.   Letting go occurs when anger gives way to more realistic expectations of your situation. You no longer expect the person with the disease to think and act "normally." You begin to adjust your lifestyle to suit the demands of the disease. You realize that the disease is not in your control and that the future is uncertain. You also no longer insist on imposing your personal wishes on reality and begin to recognize your personal limitations. One husband summed up his view in this way:

> Alzheimer's will definitely change your whole life, and your attitude has to change with it. It forces you to consider the other person's needs in front of your own. I can't see it any other way. She doesn't deserve this and you can't condemn her for it. She can't help what she has, so I have to change my life to support her. It's the agreement we made when we got married.

Acceptance.   Acceptance finally takes place when the difficult task of letting go is complete. You no longer wish to return to the past and are able to take each day at a time. Though you may not understand why this disease has come into your life, you accept it as part of your unfolding life story. Acceptance does not mean defeat, but it means taking life on its own terms. After describing a series of ups and downs in coming to terms with her husband's disease, one woman advises, "Don't be afraid to reach out and get the support you need. Just take each day as it comes and don't try to think too much about the future. If you dwell on how the person may be later on, you won't be able to enjoy their company today."

Bear in mind that you do not pass through these stages of grief all at once. Grief is resolved gradually, sometimes in fits and starts. There are too many small, successive changes and losses inherent in AD for you to be able to reach acceptance once and for all. Whenever you attain a measure of acceptance, another incident may occur that may set off another wave of grief. It is important at these trying times not to lose sight of the progress you have already made. Having a close relative, friend, counselor, or support group to guide you and remind you of your progress may ease your transition through the difficult stages of grief.

INDIVIDUAL AND FAMILY COUNSELING

In the course of caring for a loved one with AD, you may occasionally feel the need for a confidante with whom to share private thoughts and feelings. If the person with AD was your confidante in the past, then someone else must now fill this role, perhaps a close friend or relative. Sometimes a formal relationship with a nonjudgmental and objective outsider, such as a counseling professional, may be preferable.

Counseling is a valuable but often misunderstood resource. One obstacle to counseling is the stigma attached to seeking professional help for personal difficulties. Unfortunately, some people cling to the notion that they must "go it alone" and "be strong" in spite of overwhelming circumstances. Self-sufficiency and privacy are highly regarded values in our culture and can sometimes get in the way of reaching out for help. Yet knowing your limits and recognizing your need for help may actually be a positive step forward in accepting the disease. Potential benefits of engaging in a one-to-one counseling relationship include the following:

- Developing better means of handling crisis situations

- Addressing your grief

- Learning to balance your needs with the needs of the person with AD

- Improving your communication with other relatives and friends

- Discovering your inner resources

- Exploring the use of community resources

Families may also benefit from counseling. There is rarely a fair or equal division of responsibility within families in the care of a loved one with AD. Each family member copes in his or her unique way and chooses a measure of responsibility. One person typically assumes the primary role of leader on behalf of the person with AD. Others may help out in a secondary or supportive role. Still others may rarely or never get involved. Differences of opinion about decisions affecting the person with AD are bound to arise. There is much potential for conflict, especially if the role of the leader has not been fully accepted by others. One son notes, "I think families have to work hard to stay close when dealing with this disease. In our family, everybody has an opinion about what to do and how to do it." A group meeting, facilitated by a counselor and involving all concerned individuals, may help a family achieve a consensus on key issues.

Spouses and adult children may not be the only ones who are emotionally invested in decisions affecting the person with AD—grandchildren, in-laws, nieces, nephews, and close friends may also have a part to play and should be included in important decisions. One daughter-in-law commented:

> My husband and I spend most of our free time looking after his father who has Alzheimer's. My husband's three siblings live

nearby but cannot seem to accept what's going on with their father and are minimally involved with him. It took me a long time to get over the resentment I felt toward them.

A skilled counselor can facilitate discussion among all concerned parties with the goal of building a consensus. It must be kept in mind that each family has its own unique history and style of handling problems. Old conflicts unrelated to the specific issues presented by AD have a way of reemerging in stressful times, and a counselor can help everyone to focus on current issues as much as possible.

Many types of professionals are trained to provide individual and family counseling. Social workers, psychologists, psychiatrists, nurses, and pastoral counselors are employed in a variety of settings from mental health agencies to churches. They may use different approaches and techniques in helping you and others to regain a sense of equilibrium in your lives. Some professionals prefer a traditional, long-term therapy approach, while most others use short-term therapy to focus on solutions to specific issues. Time-limited and problem-focused counseling may be all you need for now.

In choosing a qualified counselor, it is advisable to get a recommendation or to check out credentials. Most professionals engaged in counseling are licensed by the state and accredited through professional organizations. Many counseling services are partially covered by health insurance, and most nonprofit agencies offer a sliding scale for fees. Virtually every county or local community provides financial support to a health or social service agency that offers counseling or makes referrals to counselors in private practice.

EXPLORING SPIRITUAL RESOURCES

Spirituality may be the least talked about but most commonly explored option among those who have primary responsibility of caring for loved ones with AD. It is in difficult times that the following questions about faith, hope, and God often come into sharp focus:

- "Why is this happening?"

- "Why do bad things happen to good people?"

- "How can God allow this to happen to me? To us?"

- "Is there a God after all?"

- "What does my religion say about this kind of trial?"

Life's difficulties have a way of intensifying a hunger within us for understanding, strength, and answers to such profound questions. Just as it has been said "There are no atheists in foxholes," spiritual issues often come to the fore among those caring for someone with AD. The search for meaning in the midst of personal confusion seems almost inevitable. For example, in *Tears in God's Bottle,* Wayne Ewing writes eloquently about how his wife's AD afforded him "an education in the wisdom of the soul."[9]

Those unaccustomed to spiritual quests may struggle with preconceived notions about God or the tenets of organized religion. And those who are on a spiritual journey may still feel shaken in their beliefs about and relationship with God. Sharon Fish, whose mother had AD, writes of how she experienced spiritual disillusionment until she could sort out her feelings: "I was very angry with God. My primary support system had always been my church. I stopped going. The Bible has always been my point of strength. I stopped reading. Prayer had always been my source of encouragement. I stopped praying."[10] Yet when these obstacles can be overcome, those who pursue a deeper spirituality often report a sense of inner peace that helps them persevere in the face of adversity. Stella Guidry writes, "At times, prayer is my only resource, and one that I use quite a bit. Without it, I don't know where I would be today."[11]

Group activities may afford some opportunities for spiritual reflection and growth. The most obvious resources are your church, synagogue, or mosque. If organized religion nurtures your spiritual growth, then worship services involving rituals, traditional prayers, hymns, and other forms of music may be helpful. Small groups may meet regularly to share prayers, discuss faith, and build community. Religious leaders, such as ministers, priests, or rabbis, are accustomed to addressing spiritual matters and should be consulted for their insight and experience.

Organized religion is not the only arena in which you can explore spirituality. If you are not inclined toward formal religious practice, an attractive alternative may be visiting one of the hundreds of retreat centers that have sprung up in recent years that do not have a strictly religious focus. These centers typically sponsor individual and group programs for spiritual direction and offer workshops on important issues about coping with life. They often employ counselors who serve as spiritual guides, either in the short-term or on an ongoing basis.

If getting away to pursue spiritual affairs is not possible, many solitary activities may also be useful. The following spiritual activities can be pursued alone:

▸ Practicing various types of prayer, rituals, meditation, and yoga

▸ Using books of structured prayers and other spiritual readings

▸ Reflecting on religious scriptures and other traditional writings

▸ Keeping a spiritual journal to record your thoughts and intuitions

▸ Listening to inspirational music

▸ Appreciating the mysteries of nature, art, and sacred objects

Spiritual care alone does not guarantee replenishment of personal energy or a renewed outlook on life. Paying attention to all levels—body, mind, and spirit—is essential for maintaining personal health and wholeness. However, nurturing your inner life can make a positive difference in how you perceive your outer life. Spiritual practices may help you come to terms with AD and lead to a sense of mission in your leadership role. One man caring for his wife summarized his new point of view:

I used to think that if you did right, then happiness would follow. But then Alzheimer's came along and blew that away. I
guess God had different plans so I needed to learn how to
make the best of a bad situation. I can't say that I've got this
disease down pat, but it's not as hard as I thought it could be.
My wife can still do a lot of things for herself and she doesn't
mind my help. So we are just taking one day at a time.

KEEPING A JOURNAL

There are at least a dozen books currently in print based on the
diaries of those who have cared for relatives with AD. These husbands, wives, sons, and daughters did not begin writing with the
goal of publishing. On the contrary, their daily writings served as
outlets for their thoughts and feelings about coping with the disease. The personal practice of "journaling" enabled them to
reflect on their experiences and to gain a better perspective on
their situation.

AD invariably evokes many strong feelings, and keeping such
feelings bottled up inside is unhealthy. You, too, might find it
helpful to keep a running account of your personal reactions to
the different stages of AD in a diary or private journal. No writing
experience is required, since keeping a journal is purely an exercise in becoming more aware of your thoughts and feelings and a
way to unclutter your mind. Writing also allows both your dark
and light sides to become better known to you. When you chart
your course during a stressful or confusing time, patterns typically
emerge that can help lead you to self-discovery and solutions to
problems. Your written record may also serve as a reminder of past
pitfalls to be avoided and successes to be savored.

Since keeping a journal requires some discipline, the following
are a few simple guidelines:

> ▸ A journal's most valuable quality is its complete flexi-
> bility. It is important to make it your own forum for self-
> expression. Let your inhibitions down and do not edit
> yourself. This is your private project and no one else's
> business.

▸ Where and when you write must fit into your lifestyle. If you can write during periods of stress, then do so. If not, wait for when you feel less distracted.

▸ The tools you use do not matter as long as they are right for you. Use a pen, pencil, spiral notebook, typewriter, word processor, or computer—whatever works for you. Keep things simple to make writing as easy and satisfying as possible.

▸ Beginning the process is probably the biggest step. Keeping a journal may develop into a pleasurable routine after a month or two. Ten minutes a day may be a good place to start.

MAINTAINING A SENSE OF HUMOR

Numerous studies have shown that humor can go a long way toward alleviating stress. Good fun, laughter, and play are effective tools in coping with the pressures of caring for someone with AD. You may think, "What's so funny about Alzheimer's?" and this is a fair question to ask, since on most levels it's no laughing matter. But much of the distress associated with a situation is related to how it is perceived. Taking a lighthearted view can alter the meaning of a situation and make all the difference in coping. Juanita Tucker writes about the need to see the brighter side in relation to her husband's AD:

> I have gone through days filled with concern and confusion as well as aggravation and anger. But I have learned to be flexible, to sort out what is really important, to keep my sense of humor. For example, one evening I was so insistent that Allan put on his pajamas at bedtime. "One doesn't sleep in shorts and a T-shirt!" I said. With a look of resignation he finally put on his pajamas. He then looked at me with a puzzled expression and asked, in all seriousness, "Is this written down somewhere?" One's priorities do have a way of changing after these funny encounters.[12]

A man I know, whose wife has AD, constantly tells jokes as a way of easing tension. He once remarked, "My wife has gotten preoccupied with the hereafter since she developed this disease." "How so?" I asked. "Well," he said, "whenever she walks into a room, she'll stand there a minute, then say 'What am I here after?'" Such humor may not appeal to everyone, but it seems to work well for him.

It is also important to spend time with friends who remind you not to get completely caught up in your troubles and to laugh now and then. One woman notes, "I have a group of lady friends that has socialized together for more than thirty years. Those women remind me how to laugh, even when I'm feeling down about my husband having Alzheimer's." In support groups for the relatives and friends of people with AD, a topic discussed in the next chapter, humor is a staple of virtually every meeting.

There is a child within each of us who can remember how to enjoy life under any circumstances. It takes a conscious choice to seek this perspective. When Gail Sheehy was doing background work for her best-selling book, *Pathfinders,* she discovered that the ability to see humor in difficult situations was a primary way for people to cope with change and uncertainty.[13] She referred to those who could successfully deal with life's crises as "pathfinders." In a real sense, family members and friends who learn to negotiate the challenges of AD are pathfinders too.

As the disease progresses, increasing amounts of time and energy will be required of you and others in caring for your loved one with AD. As the leader, you may be especially vulnerable to the stress that comes with this major responsibility. You must take steps to care for yourself in order to remain physically, mentally, and spiritually strong over the long haul. It will sometimes be necessary to call on outside sources for help so that you can nurture yourself regularly. In the next chapter, I will address some forms of help that you may need in the future, as the disease progresses.

CHAPTER 12

Obtaining the Help You May Need

> We have prepared for the worst
> and now we are planning to live
> expecting the best. If the worst
> comes, we are ready for it. If it
> doesn't, we will have not wasted
> today worrying about it.

Betty Davis, as quoted in Robert Davis's
My Journey into Alzheimer's Disease

Now is the time, in the early stages, for you and other loved ones of the person with AD to learn to pace yourselves. Caring for someone with AD over the long haul is analogous to running a marathon. Sprinting from the start will ruin your chances of completing the race, and so pacing yourself is necessary. For example, some family members and friends panic upon hearing the diagnosis of AD and eagerly start trying to absorb whatever they can about the disease. Although gaining knowledge can sometimes help you to get a handle on the situation, drowning yourself in information can be counterproductive, as you may become unduly worried or sad.

It is possible that the early stages of AD may last for many years—or the disease may progress more quickly. You cannot be sure what the future holds, and preparing for every contingency is both practically unrealistic and emotionally draining. It is helpful, to a limited degree, to understand what might happen over the next five or ten years. At the same time, you cannot allow yourself now to feel overwhelmed by the issues that you might face at the later stages of the disease, especially since it is impossible for you to imagine how you might feel and think then. This chapter focuses first on services you might need in the near term and then addresses the usual progression of AD. This book does not address issues related to the later stages of the disease. However, numerous other books, pamphlets, and videos, many of which are listed in the Resources, cover more advanced care issues.

USING COMMUNITY RESOURCES

Nearly everyone involved in directly caring for someone with AD feels the need for help at one point or another. You should not aim to be an exception—no medals are awarded to those who struggle alone. Unfortunately, seeking outside help is often seen as a personal failure or inadequacy. It is a major step to realize that your own resources may not be sufficient to provide for all the needs of the person with AD. You feel that you know exactly what the person with AD needs and how to meet those needs. However, committing yourself to caring for someone does not automatically mean that you will render all aspects of care. On the contrary, your commitment entails ensuring a good quality of life by all available means, regardless of who is actually providing the care. Therefore, you should always feel free to call upon other people and services for assistance, as long as you retain overall responsibility or share it with others. Some of the supplemental types of help that are worth considering are support groups, in-home care, and adult day services.

Most community resources are geared to the needs of individuals and families dealing with the middle and late stages of AD. Unfortunately, up to now there has been little appreciation within the service sector about the unique problems posed by the early stages. Therefore, it may take a while to find a good match between the particular needs of your loved one with AD and community resources. Persist in seeking organizations and individuals that are appropriate to your situation. It is also a good idea to enlist others in your search for the right types of help.

PARTICIPATING IN A SUPPORT GROUP

In Chapter 10 we discussed the help that support groups can offer your loved one with AD. Early-stage support groups for relatives and friends can also be helpful to you and others directly or indirectly involved in providing care, but most support groups are not limited to early-stages issues. Support groups serve two basic purposes. First, they aim to educate families and friends about the many aspects of AD. Second, they enable members to offer emotional support to one another. For the most part these groups attract people dealing with the middle and late stages of AD. For this reason, participating in a support group may have limited value for you unless the group's leader makes an effort to balance the needs of all members.

Support groups typically consist of about eight to twenty people and are led by a health-care professional or an experienced family member. The group leader is responsible for facilitating, keeping order, and focusing on the needs for education and emotional support. Meetings ordinarily last about two hours and are held monthly. Membership is usually free, and members can drop in and out at will. Some groups are structured with specific goals and agendas in mind, but most groups are conducted in an informal, conversational style.

The self-help philosophy is central to the functioning of most support groups. Members have a chance to share their collective wisdom by exchanging stories about caring for someone with AD. The operating principle is that one single perspective on the disease is less helpful than having the different perspectives of many group members. Members also share information about the symptoms of AD, how to handle communication difficulties, and how to find appropriate help such as paid companions, adult day care, or residential care. Outside speakers are occasionally invited to address topics of interest such as legal and financial planning.

Some topics discussed in support groups may be premature for newcomers to the disease. Stories about potential symptoms and experiences may be distressing to those caring for someone in the early stages of AD. Nevertheless, an effective group leader protects newcomers against undue worry about the future. The knowledge, experience, and skill of leaders can vary from group to group. If you do not receive the help you need after a meeting or two, consider joining another group or returning to the group later.

Learning about the disease in a support group does not take place only on an intellectual level. Rather, sharing feelings in a safe and confidential atmosphere enables members to realize that they are not alone. Every imaginable thought and feeling is fair game for discussion in a group, which can be a liberating experience. You can freely discuss the dilemma of caring for someone with AD while protecting your own needs without embarrassment or fear of criticism. You may get a great deal of comfort and hope from meeting others who are coping well under similar circumstances. One daughter notes, "It's important to find other people to talk to about the various problems of the disease. It's also good to get help in learning how to be more patient and understanding with the person who has the Alzheimer's."

Because of the range of different needs and circumstances of those who care for people with AD, many specialized support groups have started to spring up. For example, some groups are geared exclusively to spouses and other groups are just for adult children. Groups devoted specifically to the early stages of the disease may also be available. These specialized groups enable participants to establish rapport quickly by virtue of their similar concerns.

Although support groups alone cannot give you all the education and emotional support needed to deal with AD, they can be a valuable source of help. Indeed, for some people who lack a solid network of relatives and friends, support groups have proven to be a real lifeline. To find out about support groups in your area, contact the local chapter of the Alzheimer's Association ([800] 272-3900) or the Alzheimer Society of Canada ([800] 616-8816).

Many hospitals, adult day centers, and social service agencies also sponsor support groups.

For those who cannot or do not wish to venture into traditional support groups, the Internet affords a way to be in contact with others without leaving your home. Public-service organizations and commercial enterprises have formed groups through the Internet to help people with common interests to communicate easily with one another. These so-called news groups, bulletin boards, and chat rooms enable group members to provide information and support to one another based on their mutual interests. One on-line group with over a thousand members concerned specifically with AD is maintained by the Alzheimer's Disease Research Center at Washington University in St. Louis. For information about how to participate in this informative group, see the Internet Resources. Similar groups devoted to AD are also available through Internet providers such as America Online, CompuServe, Prodigy Internet, and the Microsoft Network.

USING HELP AT HOME

At first, most people in the early stages of the disease can be left alone at home without much worry about their well-being and safety. However, you or your loved one with AD will gradually begin to wonder if being alone is a good idea. There may be growing limits to his or her ability to be self-directed and feel comfortable at home alone. You will eventually realize that supervision is needed some of the time, and then ultimately at all times, in order to reduce worry—yours and your loved one's. Whether such help is needed on a part-time, full-time, or live-in basis is primarily your decision and will depend on many factors, including affordability. It is not realistic for you to be available on a continuous basis, 24 hours a day, seven days a week. Nobody can handle all the responsibilities involved in caring for someone with AD alone, nor should such heroics be attempted. If care is to continue indefinitely at home, it will be necessary for you to get regular breaks.

It takes courage to reach out, but you and your loved one with AD stand to benefit from the help of other people. You may initially prefer to call upon your relatives, neighbors, and friends. They may fill in gaps or be available on a regular basis, but you must overcome a natural tendency to believe that they will somehow just understand what is needed and when it is needed. You may need to assert yourself and ask for specific types of assistance at specific times. Even with the help of one or more supportive persons, you may need to consider hiring additional help. You may be able to work out a paid arrangement with someone you know so that the helper's personal commitment is bolstered by a financial incentive. Do not hesitate to consider such a business proposition with someone you know, since the alternative of hiring someone through an agency can be risky. Volunteer services may also be available in some areas, so this avenue should be explored. Many religious congregations have formed volunteer groups to assist individuals in need of part-time care. You can contact Faith in Action, an interfaith volunteer program, by calling toll-free (877) 324-8411, or contact Shepherd's Centers of America by calling (800) 547-7073, to see if there is a program in your area.

Bringing a stranger into the home to care for the person with AD can be a big gamble, so this option is usually not considered until it becomes essential. Worries about having an outsider in the home cannot be easily dismissed. When you are the chief provider of care, you can count on your own reliability, sensitivity, and honesty. As soon as you share responsibility with others, especially a paid helper, these concerns can no longer be guaranteed. Myriad troubling questions arise. Will the helper show up on time? Will he or she be patient and kind? Might she or he be trustworthy, patronizing, or worse, a thief? Yet, although there are indeed risks involved in bringing a paid helper into the home, the risks of not getting help may be even bigger. And there may be unexpected benefits if you hire someone who meets or exceeds your expectations. This kind of arrangement can prove successful for everyone if the right person is found for the job.

You can hire someone either privately or through a home-care agency, and there are advantages and disadvantages to either approach. On the one hand, you benefit by having a direct choice instead of settling for whoever is sent by an agency. You can be selective and set your own standards. The expense of a private arrangement is also far less than using an agency. You can negotiate an hourly, daily, or weekly rate rather than paying a higher rate set by an agency. On the other hand, there are also several drawbacks to a private arrangement. Unemployment, Social Security, and Medicare taxes are supposed to be paid on behalf of your employee if payments exceed one thousand dollars a year. If a paid helper gets sick or quits, you are not guaranteed an instant replacement.

Home-care agencies provide an array of services on a fee-for-service basis, and offer several levels of staff. A "companion," homemaker, or nursing assistant may be well suited to providing most services you need. Turnover tends to be a big problem at home-care agencies as well as in private arrangements. However, an agency can usually provide a substitute or replacement within a short time. The hassles for you of screening, interviewing, and hiring the right person for the job may outweigh the financial benefits. Yet there is no guarantee that someone hired through an agency will be any better qualified than someone you hire privately. For additional tips about hiring a helper, I recommend the guidebook *Hiring Home Caregivers* listed in the Resources.

Since virtually all the care provided at home to someone with AD is not covered by Medicare or other forms of insurance, with the exception of long-term-care insurance, out-of-pocket expenses can be quite high. Rates range from $12 to $20 an hour, up to $175 for one entire day. As noted in Chapter 9, the cost of hiring someone to perform medical, maintenance, and personal care services should qualify as an itemized tax deduction under federal law, provided that all medical expenses exceed 7.5 percent of adjusted gross income in a given year. Whether the services are considered "medical" depends on the nature of the services performed and not on the qualifications of the person performing them. If a paid helper performs both medical and housekeeping services such as dressing, grooming, and bathing, only the medical portion is considered tax deductible. If the expense of hiring someone does not qualify as medical care as defined by the Internal Revenue Service, it may still qualify for the Household and

Dependent Care Credit if the person with AD resides with you. Government subsidies for services provided by home-care agencies under contract with state-funded programs might be available to people with low incomes and few assets. Contact the Eldercare Locator ([800] 677-1116) for further information about programs and eligibility requirements in your state.

Although cost is an important consideration, distrust of strangers and concern about the quality of care are the most common barriers to using in-home services. You can take the following steps to ensure that risks are kept to a minimum when working with an agency:

Identify needs. What type of services are needed—companionship, meal preparation, dressing, bathing? A job description that fits the particular needs of the person with AD should be written down and discussed with a prospective agency or employee. If you want your loved one to be an active participant in activities with a paid helper or a passive recipient of services, then the nature of the job should be clarified. Also, a schedule showing the days and hours that you need covered in a given week should be organized. Home-care agencies usually require that you hire a helper for a minimum of four hours a day. If you are uncertain about how often to have your helper come, at least twice a week is a good start.

Make your own selection of an agency and helper. Obtain a list of agencies that are known to specialize in caring for people with AD. Ask for referrals from the local chapter of the Alzheimer's Association, the state agency on aging, or discharge planners at nearby hospitals. A good agency promptly returns calls, carefully listens to requests, and provides written details about services and costs. You should discuss your specific needs and expectations with the agency *and* the paid helper, since it cannot be assumed that the agency has communicated details to the helper. If possible, conduct an interview with the prospective helper to inquire about his or her training, experience, and references. A background check of past criminal history should also be done by the agency. Above all, look for personal qualities such as patience, understanding, a sense of humor, and good personal chemistry with your loved one with AD.

Develop a working relationship with the helper. A paid helper deserves to be given clear instructions and immediate feedback, both positive and negative. Pass along the benefits of your experience by teaching the helper what works and what doesn't work in relation to your loved one with AD. Make concrete suggestions, provide encouragement, and ask clarifying questions. Consider sharing educational resources with your helper to increase his or her knowledge about the disease. It may take several visits by the helper before everyone involved settles into a routine.

Evaluate progress. Evaluation should be an ongoing process, but regular times need to be set aside for discussing your concerns. Reward good work and address any problems in a straightforward manner. Difficulties are inevitable, but good communication can minimize them and yield quick solutions. Flagrant mistakes and repeated misunderstandings call for intervention by the paid helper's supervisor.

CHOOSING AN ADULT DAY CENTER

Another option to consider is adult day care, a community-based program offering therapeutic activities and individualized services in a group setting for older adults with a variety of disabilities. Most people who attend adult day centers have AD, but people with other disabilities are welcome too. Some people find the term *day care* offensive because of its association with children. More adult terms like *day center* or *club* may be more appealing to people with AD, who rightfully do not wish to be treated like children.

Those attending adult day centers can participate in structured recreational activities under the direction of a professional staff. The daily schedule of activities includes nutritious meals and snacks. Some centers also provide transportation, dispense medications, and assist with personal tasks such as bathing. People with AD typically enjoy the opportunity to be with other people in a place where their needs and abilities are understood.

Adult day centers may be a good option to consider when one or more of the conditions listed below are present. The person with AD

▸ appears unable to provide him- or herself with any structure for daily activities.

▸ is isolated from others for more than a few hours a day and misses companionship.

▸ cannot be safely left alone at home.

▸ lives with someone who works outside the home or needs regular time away from home for other reasons.

The ideal is to find an adult day center that is the right fit for the affected person's needs. You may even have the luxury of choosing from more than one place close to home. Centers tend to offer similar services, but some cater exclusively to those with AD. For the most part, though, participants are in the middle and late stages of the disease. At present, relatively few adult day centers have specialized programs for people in the early stages of AD.

There are many ways to approach the decision to involve your loved one with AD in an adult day center. First and foremost, you must be comfortable with the idea. You may imagine that the person with AD would probably not like it, but you need to keep an open mind. Staff at these centers usually welcome exploratory visits, and you may be surprised at the friendliness of the setting. Two daughters reluctantly brought their mother to a center one day, convinced that she would reject the idea of participation after an introductory visit. They claimed that she had never been a "joiner" and was too proud to be around others with memory problems. While the daughters met with one staff member, other staff invited their mother into a group activity. When they reunited an hour later, the daughters were surprised by their mother's reaction: "I like this place. The people here are forgetful like me and yet nobody is expected to remember. They have nice people here who help keep you on track."

When discussing this option with the person with AD, it is best to use a positive, calm, and reassuring manner. Simple and brief explanations, such as, "It's a place where you can meet some friendly people" or "The doctor thinks you should try this out so I think it's worth checking out too" are most effective. Most people with AD will follow this type of suggestion if you set the right tone from the beginning. Some people with AD, like the mother mentioned above, react well to their first visit to an adult day center; others are put off by the unfamiliar situation. The staff at these centers have a lot of experience with this and know how to ease the adjustment. Some staff even make home visits to get to know prospective participants. It is customary to try out the adult day center two or three times a week at first and then to increase the frequency of visits as the person's comfort level grows. Although your loved one may express some resistance initially, allow the trial to continue for a few weeks. The payoff comes when the person with AD begins to feel safe and to enjoy the company of other participants and staff.

Most centers are open five days a week and some are open on Saturdays as well. The cost is roughly $50 a day. In the United States, Medicare does not cover the cost, so most people have to pay out of their own pocket. However, the cost should qualify as an itemized tax deduction for medical expenses under federal law, provided that all medical expenses exceed 7.5 percent of adjusted gross income in a given year. Again, if the expense does not qualify for this type of tax deduction, it may still qualify for the Household and Dependent Care Credit if the person with AD resides with you.

Financial assistance for those with low incomes and few assets may be available through public sources such as the state Department on Aging or the U.S. Department of Veterans Affairs. A sliding-fee scale may also be available at some centers for those people ineligible for subsidies. Discounts are usually allowed for people who attend daily.

Information about local adult day centers can be obtained through a hospital social worker, nurse, or physician. The National Adult Day Services Association, which can be reached toll-free at (866) 890-7357, maintains an extensive listing of centers. Information about the local centers as well as other services can be obtained directly from your state's department on aging or through the Eldercare Locator at (800) 677-1116.

THE NATIONAL FAMILY CAREGIVER SUPPORT PROGRAM

The U.S. government enacted an important new program in 2000, known as the National Family Caregiver Support Program, to assist families who care for older disabled adults, including those with AD. Whether or not you consider yourself to be a caregiver, this program may benefit you now or in the future. The program is administered by the Administration on Aging of the U.S. Department of Health and Human Services. The Administration on Aging works with a network of national, state, and local organizations to plan, coordinate, and provide home and community-based services. Most of the funds from this national program are allocated to states based on their proportional share of the population aged 70 years and older. The program is administered locally by private, nonprofit organizations or government entities known as area agencies on aging (AAAs), which contract with community-service providers to offer the following five basic services:

1. Information about available services

2. Assistance in gaining access to supportive services

3. Individual counseling, organization of support groups, and training to assist caregivers in making decisions and solving problems

4. Respite care to enable caregivers to be temporarily relieved from caregiving responsibilities

5. Supplemental services to complement the care provided by caregivers

Your local AAA should be among the first resources contacted for information about these and other useful services. Priority consideration is given to persons in the greatest social and economic need, but there are no income or asset limits for eligi-

bility. Local AAAs are generally listed in the city or county government sections of the telephone directory under "Aging" or
"Social Services." You can also find out about services in your
local area by contacting the Eldercare Locator at (800) 677-1116.

LEARNING MORE ABOUT AD

You may not want or need the types of services described above
while your loved one is in the early stages of AD. Nevertheless,
worsening symptoms over time may make the use of additional
resources necessary.

The challenges of the disease right now may be more than
enough for you to handle without worrying about the future, yet
you may be curious about what may lie ahead. If current challenges are handled well, there is reason to believe that your self-
confidence will grow as you face the challenges ahead. Exercise
caution in anticipating these changes, though, since planning for
every contingency is not possible. Nevertheless, you and others
involved in day-to-day responsibilities should have some idea of
the changes that accompany AD, so that you can prepare accordingly.

Table 12.1 (see page 230) gives an overview of typical symptoms at the early, middle, and late stages of AD.[1] Note that these
three stages are not clear-cut, and symptoms frequently overlap.
The continuum from complete independence to total dependence
may take anywhere from three to twenty years. Most people can be
cared for at home for the major part of the disease, and relocating
them to a nursing home is not inevitable. Furthermore, many people with AD never reach the late stages of the disease but die from
other illnesses before reaching a point of total dependence. As
symptoms worsen, there will be a corresponding increase in the
amount of help needed by the person with the disease.

Generally speaking, the more troubling symptoms that sometimes occur in the later stages of AD are the ones that receive the
most attention in popular descriptions of the disease. The media
tend to focus on worst-case scenarios. However, problems such
as aggressive behavior, wandering, hallucinations, insomnia, and

incontinence do not occur in all cases. If and when these problems occur, they may be triggered by many causes, such as a drug reaction or an acute illness. These problems may seriously affect the quality of life for everyone directly involved and deserve the close attention of professionals. Do not hesitate to call upon others for help if these problems arise.

Table 12.1: Stages and Symptoms of Alzheimer's Disease

Note: These stages are not clearly defined and symptoms often overlap.

	Early Stage	Middle Stage	Late Stage
1. Memory	Frequent loss of recent memory	Persistent loss of recent memory	Confusion about past and present memory time
2. Language	Mild aphasia (difficulty expressing and comprehending)	Moderate aphasia	Severe aphasia
3. Orientation	Potential to get lost in unfamiliar places	Potential to get lost in familiar places	Misidentification of familiar people and places
4. Motor Control	Some difficulty writing, using objects	Slowed walking	Possible falls, possible immobility
5. Mood and Behavior	Possible apathy, depression	Possible mood and behavioral disturbances	Greater incidence of mood and behavioral disturbances
6. Activities of Daily Living (ADLs)	Need for reminders with some ADLs	Need for reminders and help with most ADLs	Need for help with all ADLs

(*Source: Adapted with permission from D. Kuhn, "The Normative Crises of Families Confronting Dementia,"* Families in Society: The Journal of Contemporary Human Services 71, no. 8 (1990): 451–60.)

Over the past decade, there has been a virtual flood of information about AD produced by both professionals and family members of people with AD. Some of the more helpful resources are listed at the end of this book. Books, pamphlets, videos, and information found on the Internet abound, but the quality of this information varies widely. The tone in some materials is rather negative in that there is a tendency to dwell on the growing inability of the person with AD and the burden on families. Grim images of individuals and families struggling to survive the "funeral that never ends" can be misleading and frightening. It takes a strong will and heart to hear and read about the full gamut of possibilities and not feel overwhelmed. Seek reliable and balanced information as needed. Pessimistic stories abound but there are many positive stories of hope, love, and meaning associated with caring for someone with AD. Stay informed, but do not give up hope that a good quality of life is possible for everyone involved.

Another disadvantage of the literally thousands of books, articles, and webpages devoted to topics such as diagnosis, genetics, treatments, alternative medicine, and coping strategies for AD is that although you may find some of this material useful, you may soon become overwhelmed. As one person noted, "At first I tried to get my hands on everything about this disease, but I ended up getting more confused and upset. Now I advise others to stop reading about Alzheimer's and start coping day-by-day. I know this approach has worked for me."

Your own expectations for finding enjoyment in life, now and in the future, will naturally be tempered by your loved one's disease, but keep in mind that personal fulfillment and meaning are still possible. Indeed, a more positive outlook may develop as valuing each day and living in the moment become a growing reality. Changing your attitude and behavior to accommodate the presence of AD in your life doesn't happen overnight. Nothing less than major lifestyle changes are called for, a process that takes time. Along the way, your progress in making adjustments may feel painstakingly slow. Mistakes are inevitable in the course of learning how to cope effectively with your changing roles and responsibilities. Do not be discouraged by setbacks. Such disappointments are also opportunities to learn new skills and redefine what constitutes a good life.

A wise woman whose husband had AD once told me, "The human spirit is like a tea bag: You don't know your own strength until you've been in hot water." AD will certainly test you in all kinds of ways. Although the disease cannot be stopped or reversed, you will always have the freedom to choose how you cope with its challenges. May you discover surprising strength within your own spirit.

. . . .
                .
                .
                .

CHAPTER 13

Voices of Experience

*As we cultivate peace and
happiness in ourselves, we also
nourish peace and happiness in
those we love.*

Thich Nhat Hanh

Relatives and friends of people with AD have published at least a hundred books about their experiences of caring for someone with the disease. Although each story is unique, these books can offer you guidance through the maze of AD. Some of the better ones are listed in the Resources under each chapter's heading.

This chapter will highlight the experience of family members and friends of people with AD who completed a survey that I developed specifically for this chapter. I wanted to hear directly from those who have cared for loved ones with AD so you could learn from them. The survey was sent to them with the cooperation of my professional colleagues working at AD research centers and other AD service programs throughout the United States and Canada. Within a month, I received nearly two hundred replies from husbands, wives, sons, daughters, daughters-in-law, sons-in-laws, siblings, and close friends. Their combined experience caring for someone with AD totals over 1,400 years, an average of seven years per person since the diagnosis. Virtually all of them have loved ones who have progressed into the later stages of AD. I did not inquire about their racial, ethnic, and cultural back-grounds so they are not necessarily a representative group. I suspect that since they are interested in sharing their experience with others, for the most part they have adapted fairly well to caring for a relative with AD. Your experience may or may not be represented by them, although some of their thoughts and feelings may parallel your own.

While some individuals offered short, simple responses to a series of open-ended questions, others wrote lengthy explanations and anecdotes. Some people wrote in straightforward, factual terms, while most told of an emotion-filled experience, often referred to as a "journey." Most were either older individuals themselves or were middle-aged people caring for older people. In a few cases, the individuals with AD were middle-aged and their spouses were respondents. Most people are still caring for someone at home, some care for others who now live in residential care facilities, and a few had experienced the death of a loved one with AD within the past year. Whereas some clearly appear angry and depressed, most have reached a measure of hard-fought accept-ance. Their similarities and differences will be illustrated through a question and answer format.

QUESTIONS AND ANSWERS

Q *When you first heard the diagnosis of Alzheimer's disease, what was your initial reaction? How did your thoughts and feelings about the disease change over time?*

About half of the people report that the diagnosis was a total shock. Feelings of denial, disbelief, anger, fear, and sadness were common at first. The notion of AD as "the worst possible disease" was a typical reaction to the news. One woman writes, "Upon hearing the diagnosis, I thought my whole world would fall apart. It felt as if my husband had been handed a death sentence." A few people say they ignored the diagnosis, not talking about it or doing anything in response for weeks or months afterwards. A wife writes, "After a few weeks, I collected my senses and began to rearrange our future plans." Getting the proper information and support generally enabled them to cope with difficult feelings and develop positive coping strategies. A husband notes, "At first I was devastated. For about six months we did nothing in response. After a respectful period of pondering, we got involved in research projects, support groups, and many other activities related to Alzheimer's." Getting a realistic understanding about the nature of AD was essential for coping with the shock experienced at the beginning. A son writes, "Since I have a close friend whose mother is in the late stages of Alzheimer's, I was horrified contemplating Mom's future. But then I began to realize that it can be a lengthy process and people can function pretty well for a long time. I switched my attitude and found ways to help her."

For the other half, who had expected to hear the diagnosis, an evaluation confirmed what they already had suspected for months or years beforehand. For many of these individuals, the label "Alzheimer's disease" provided insight into the symptoms and gave them a framework for better understanding. A wife writes, "At least I finally knew what was causing his unusual behavior and could learn how to make adjustments." The diagnosis also enabled them to talk openly about the disease and to be proactive about decisions that needed to be made. A daughter writes, "It was sad to know that my mother had struggled with this alone prior to being diagnosed. We knew something was wrong but pretended it would go away. The diagnosis gave us a way to bring it out into the open."

Although some people report being intellectually prepared to hear the diagnosis, it nevertheless evoked feelings of grief as thoughts turned to feelings of loss and worry about a loved one's decline. Again, the implications of the diagnosis were generally unknown and most could only imagine a dreadful future. A daughter writes, "Over time, we've come to understand the implications and impact of the disease on both our family and my mother." A wife notes, "It was helpful to know that it is a disease which, though predictable in many ways[,] is very individual in the way it alters the person's thinking and behavior. I learned to be observant as to how it affected him specifically and that helped me determine how to help him."

Q *At the time of diagnosis, did the doctor or another professional say or do anything particularly helpful or unhelpful?*

Several people report that obtaining a proper evaluation and diagnosis from a physician was in itself a major struggle. Their complaints about a loved one's poor memory were often unheeded or attributed simply to "old age." A couple of people recall being dismissed by physicians who coldly remarked that nothing could be done about memory loss. A woman reflects back on that time: "I am still angry about the doctor's pessimism. I have since learned that there is so much you can do and little of it has to do with medicine." Other people report getting only a vague diagnosis at first and their lingering uncertainty about the condition proved frustrating. On the other hand, many people tell of getting proper yet incomplete attention from physicians. Seldom were they encouraged to obtain a second opinion or seek out a professional well versed in caring for someone with AD. If dissatisfied with a primary care physician, specialists were typically sought out and found to be good sources of help.

Physicians were generally knowledgeable about antidementia medications. A prescription was usually written for one of the AD drugs, and potential benefits and side effects were briefly discussed. Medical issues were addressed but the myriad social and psychological issues of the disease were ignored for the most part. One woman complained that although the doctor called her adult son to discuss the diagnosis, her key role as a spouse of someone with AD was overlooked. In most cases, the impact of the disease on relatives and friends was not foremost in physicians' minds.

Apart from those at memory disorder clinics or AD research centers, very few physicians offered to convene a meeting of concerned relatives and friends. In those special cases, physicians answered questions, shared printed materials, and made referrals to community resources. Family members share universal appreciation for straight facts, realistic advice, and warm concern. A daughter in-law reflects, "The doctor made a point of saying that there was life after a diagnosis. That positive message has stayed with our family and has challenged us to make the most of the situation." A husband tells of his gratitude for the doctor's emphasis on the slowness of the disease and the fact that there was time to enjoy many things with his wife. He remarks, "I appreciated the doctor's honesty that my wife and I were now living on borrowed time together. It helped me realize the urgency in making the most of this bad situation."

Q *As you look back at the time of the diagnosis, what would have been more helpful?*

Some people report satisfaction with physicians but most expressed concern that physicians did not adequately prepare them for either the short-term or long-term consequences of AD. A wife notes, "I would have benefited from more aggressive follow-up. I got the impression that a one-shot consultation was the doctor's modus operandi." Family members did not expect physicians to address all of their issues and were relatively forgiving because of the physician's busy schedule. At the same time, they clearly needed ongoing support, education, and services and were generally not directed to resources. One husband observes, "Physicians know little about the day-to-day care of people with this disease. I had to make do on my own until I got connected to the right people." To help him cope with his wife's condition, he found a social worker, a financial advisor, an attorney, and a support group. A wife says simply, "Above all, I needed reassurance that all was not lost." A daughter in-law writes, "What our family needed was a learning environment. A multi-disciplinary team would have been most helpful but I would have settled for just one mentor. It's tough to learn things on your own when you don't even know the right questions to ask." Lack of information appears to compound feelings of loneliness and desperation. A husband notes, "Having come through this initial period, I believe there is a big need to acknowledge the emotional trauma and get guidance in taking on a new role."

In light of many disappointing remarks about physicians, it is interesting to note that several research studies that have explored physician and family interactions have yielded similar findings.[1] Families facing the diagnosis of AD generally consider care by physicians to be satisfactory but less than ideal. Families consistently complain that physicians give little attention to their need for information and referral and seldom address emotional distress. A survey commissioned by the Alzheimer's Association revealed that only 124 of 376 people felt that they received all of the information they wanted from their primary care physicians.[2] Yet 440 of the 550 physicians surveyed believed that they were providing the necessary advice and recommendations. This survey illustrates a communication gap between physicians and family members. It suggests that families may not be prepared to hear what physicians are trying to convey at the time of diagnosis. It also suggests that physicians are not sensitive to the needs of families at this particularly difficult time and need to reinforce their initial advice and recommendations at follow-up appointments.

At any rate, ongoing support, education, and services are needed throughout the course of AD. Setting the right tone for the future may be the best form of help provided by physicians or other health professionals at the outset. At the same time, families must seek out additional forms of help instead of relying solely upon a single physician to address their needs related to AD.

Q *How have relatives, friends, neighbors, and others reacted to the news that someone they know has been diagnosed with Alzheimer's disease?*

Nearly all of the family members report a mixed bag—favorable reactions by some people and unfavorable reactions by others. They tell of varied reactions of acceptance and denial among relatives and friends. Some people were already aware that something was amiss, many months or, in some cases, years before the actual diagnosis. Others were completely surprised and required more time to come to terms, especially if they were not close to the situation. A spouse recalls, "At first, most friends were uncomfortable with the changes in him and I found myself in the middle as an 'interpreter.' A few chose not to see him as he had become, preferring instead to remember him the way he was." Many people agree that other relatives and friends tend to withdraw. Several individuals agree that "You find out who your friends are." Older spouses, in particular, report feeling sadness in seeing friends drift away in these trying times.

Despite such disappointments, many other individuals report that some relatives and friends manage to rise to the occasion and help out in significant ways. A woman says, "It has been gratifying to see how many people really care about us. I don't know what I would do without such a strong network of supporters." One man says he is grateful that he and his wife with AD are still treated as a couple by their friends. He notes, "They have adapted to the changes better than I had anticipated."

Q *If experienced, what is your opinion of current medications used in treating the disease?*

The majority of respondents report experience in having loved ones use the antidementia drugs. Although some indicate that side effects were intolerable, most comment favorably. At the same time, they are quick to point out that miracles are not to be expected. They caution that there is no way of really knowing if a drug is working or if the person would be the same without taking it. Most had observed an initial improvement in "alertness" or "initiative" but such benefits tapered off. If one particular drug did not seem effective or caused adverse effects, another drug was usually tried. Drugs seem to offer hope that something is being done to improve symptoms or slow the progression of AD. Several people note their concern that if an antidementia drug was discontinued, decline might result that might not have otherwise occurred.

Whether or not a medication was effective, most people believe it is an option that must be tried, at least for a while. Likewise, a minority of people indicate that supplements such as gingko biloba also must be tried despite no proven effectiveness. Overall, family members say whether drugs or supplements worked was less important than knowing that everything possible was being tried.

Q *What types of help have been most effective in planning for the future or making decisions?*

Apart from help provided by other family members and friends, most people report seeking out services to help in planning for the future. Most people note that getting legal and financial affairs in order is a top priority and therefore most had consulted a local elder-law attorney. They also report getting good information about AD and other resources at local chapters of the Alzheimer's Association or Alzheimer Society. A number of computer savvy individuals say they looked to the Internet for information and found websites and bulletin boards to be useful.

Many people say that they eventually sought out support groups and found good opportunities for information and camaraderie with others dealing with similar situations. These groups were described as vitally important in some cases. One wife says that the people in the support group give her confidence that she can face the future: "It's like being pregnant for the first time. I was petrified and thought I would not survive it. Then I thought of all those women through the ages that had survived perfectly well, so surely I would." A husband describes a deep attachment to a men's support group and drives 170 miles twice a month to participate. A few family members note that information shared in support groups is not always reliable or consistent. Some people tell of dropping out of support groups after awhile or never taking part in them at all. A few say that individual counseling on a private basis was a worthwhile investment.

Several older spouses say that the best preparation for their future involved choosing a continuing care retirement community. With several levels of care and a staff of professionals, this setting affords them permanent security as well as daily opportunities for socialization with other older adults. Moreover, they say that not having to rely on their adult children all of the time is a great relief.

Q *What has been the most challenging aspect of dealing with the disease thus far?*

Responses to this question vary from person to person. Some people focus on daily care issues such as household and personal care tasks or engaging a loved one with activities. Juggling all of these responsibilities is truly stressful in such cases. However, most people consider the emotional aspects to be most challenging. For example, overcoming denial and reaching acceptance of mental decline by a spouse or parent was seen as critical. One woman refers to the first few years of her husband's AD as "the turmoil period." A daughter-in-law notes, "Getting everyone in the family on the same page has been a cause of many heated disagreements. People clearly move at a different pace accepting the reality of Alzheimer's. The challenge is to make sure that everyone is kept well informed since emotions can get out of hand if [all family members are] not kept in the loop."

Many people describe a fine line between trying to keep the relationship as normal as possible and taking into account the changes in a loved one due to AD. A wife notes, "It's been difficult to continue participating in activities such as golf, bowling, gardening, and socializing with friends. You have to change gears often and figure out new ways to make these things continue smoothly. Sometimes you have to stop altogether." Many people describe difficulty getting other relatives and friends to understand what is happening and how to be involved. A husband says, "I needed to be specific about what I wanted from others or otherwise, they would not know. At first, I guess I expected them to read my mind. It has gotten better now that they have some direct experience of caring for my wife."

Q *What has been most useful in dealing with day-to-day care issues?*

If relatives and friends were available, their help was considered most useful. However, most people eventually tell of seeking out additional resources such as a paid helper or an adult day center. Anything done at home or at a day center to keep the person with AD positively engaged with activities or people is seen as useful. Several individuals tell of the critical role of adult day centers in giving them relief from care responsibilities and helping their relatives with AD enjoy time away from home. In addition, they say that staff members of day centers offer a wealth of information and support. A wife notes, "The women who run the day center are my angels. They have helped me keep my sanity while keeping my husband happy." Several individuals warn about "not doing this alone" and the need to get relief for one's own welfare. A man came to the following realization in relation to his wife with AD: "When she is having a bad day and I'm having a good day, life is manageable. When she is having a good day and I'm having a bad day, life is manageable too. When both of you are having bad days, then you need help." A son reports, "Once I got solid professional help, I could take charge and be proactive for a change." A wife notes, "I felt guilty at first for doing enjoyable things apart from him. I eventually learned that although he preferred me at all times, others could substitute. I would come back home feeling refreshed." A daughter notes that her mother was resistant to any form of help until an older woman was introduced as a "friend," secretly paid by the daughter.

Q *What have you found most useful in coping with your emotions over the course of the disease?*

Most people found a number of coping strategies to be useful. Most individuals describe feelings of loss and difficulty accepting changes in their relationship with the person with AD. A wife reports that her greatest difficulty was in being honest about her feelings, "especially the dark ones." Self-relaxation techniques, prayer, physical exercise, support groups, and humor were among the most commonly used ways of coping with difficult emotions. Talking with a friend or a counselor was also useful for a number of people, especially spouses. A husband notes, "Until I was able to step outside of our relationship and deal with it almost in the third person, I had a lot of sad days." For adult children who are married, having a supportive spouse is seen as invaluable for working through difficult emotions. Those who are employed often look to their jobs as a good outlet.

Many individuals write of discovering a sense of satisfaction and meaning in the current situation. This typically grows out of crisis that is resolved by reframing or renegotiating their relationship with the person with AD. A husband writes, "After I got through my deep anger, I found out how to love my wife in profoundly simple ways." A daughter says, "When I stopped looking to my dad to control himself and focused instead on understanding him, I was better able to handle my emotions." One woman looks upon her husband's AD as "a project" that she is determined to cope with successfully on a day-to-day basis. A man who practices Buddhist meditation refers to his wife's disease as the "Alzheimer's opportunity" in which both he and his wife can be transformed into their essential selves.

Q **What are you most hopeful about? Even if a cure or a treatment to stop Alzheimer's is not found soon, what keeps you going?**

Relatively few people cling to the hope for a cure or better medical treatments. The vast majority express the realization that scientific advances will not be available in time for their benefit. While generally hopeful that future generations will benefit from biomedical research, they now focus their attention on coping with everyday concerns of the caring relationship. Hope for today seems to be enough in most cases. A husband writes, "I have no hope for a medical breakthrough but what keeps me going is the love I have for my wife." A wife notes, "I think a cure will be found some day but too late for us. Meanwhile, taking one day at a time seems to work best. Every new today is mine." A daughter's goal is put simply: "I just want my dad to finish well and I am most hopeful that I can make this happen." A husband declares, "I just want to outlive my wife and see that she gets the best possible care." A wife echoes this sentiment: "I just hope that I can remain healthy and strong and see my husband right through to the end." Another wife expresses her view succinctly: "I see no hope for a cure. What keeps me going is love, pure and simple."

Others have a more philosophical outlook. A wife remarks, "I am most hopeful for a cure for our children and grandchildren. In the meantime, what keeps me going is the belief that there is a plan for my life. I accept the hand I've been dealt." A son says, "What keep me going is the certainty that I am always learning from other people and experience. Change is possible to fit any situation." A daughter adds, "I don't look for a cure or better medical treatment. I look for ways to rekindle the spirit—both hers and mine." A husband says, "I have no illusions about a miracle cure. I am most hopeful that I can look ahead now instead of looking back. This adjustment in my attitude is what enables me to take care of my wife." A son says, "I am not necessarily hopeful for a cure but for a better understanding that we can enjoy the moment and be better able to offer dignity and quality of life to older people." A daughter-in-law says, "I am hopeful that future generations won't have to face Alzheimer's. My faith keeps me going for now."

Q   *What has been the best part, if any, of caring for someone with Alzheimer's disease? In other words, has anything good come out of this experience for you?*

This question evoked perhaps the most interesting responses. A few people chose not to respond at all and another small minority indicated that the negatives outweighed the positives. For example, a wife writes, "I do not see any good coming from what I see as a slow death. But I know he would do the same for me if roles were reversed." Another wife observes, "To be honest, I don't see anything positive about this. I guess it's good that I am coping and that my husband is happy. And there will be life after Alzheimer's." A wife writes, "So far nothing but frustration has come from my husband's Alzheimer's. He's easy to talk to but he forgets everything."

However, most people write about the surprising benefits of caring for someone with AD. This experience often had resulted in an improved relationship with the person with AD or other family members and friends. Above all, this experience brought forth a personal resiliency and intense resolve that would have been unimaginable previously. The following quotes attest to the transforming nature of the care experience:

I am a better person now, more patient and tolerant, less self-centered. I am glad to help my husband who has always helped me.

Once I got in touch with my unconditional love, I took care of my wife because I wanted to and not because I had to. It has deepened my spiritual life and made me more aware of other's suffering. I have become more socially responsible.

From being part of a support group, I have learned much about devotion and loving kindness. I am grateful for the chance to meet such amazing people. They are unsung heroes and heroines.

The best part of this is knowing that our love still endures.

He relies on me for everything and sometimes I feel smothered. Yet we have grown closer. I continue to grow stronger every day on my own too. I now do things that I never dreamed possible.

Alzheimer's has lifted mother's inhibitions. Although a cause for embarrassment at times, she is now a far more happy and lovable person than in the past. I feel so blessed to have this time with her.

Now instead of fighting what fate has put before me, I can see in hindsight that I have been enriched by this experience. While cynics may think this makes me sound like Pollyanna, there have been points along this frequently dark road where I have felt blessed and rewarded. I am also satisfied knowing that I have made a positive difference in my mother-in-law's quality of life. I know she appreciates the effort too.

I have come to love my mother very deeply and to appreciate [that] her essence as a person remains and responds to love, care, humor, joy, and closeness. I have come to understand a deeper form of intimacy beyond words.

I have more fun with my dad now than I ever have. He was always doing guy stuff when I was growing up but now he's there for me to talk with about the past and laugh. I could not wire circuits with him before but now we enjoy separating Legos by color. Go figure . . . a blessing in the midst of this!

Caring for my husband has enlightened me to the depth and expanse of the strength and patience I possess, much more than I was ever aware of before being faced with this challenge. We both had the joy of family, friends, and neighbors who have been with us on this journey.

I have put aside the things that separated me from my mother—so much stuff that doesn't really matter. I have also been able to get along better with my siblings.

I have learned patience, how to listen and empathize. But it is a heck of a way to learn. I have never known so much pain.

Although I am still trying to overcome my anger and frustration, I see that we have grown closer together as a family.

My dad's disease has advanced to the degree that he no longer recognizes me but I am grateful that he feels loved. The best part is knowing that he is truly happy in spite of Alzheimer's.

It would be better if my father did not have this disease but the best thing I have found out is that my husband is a wonderful and caring son-in law.

We are now closer as an entire family as we work together to care for my mother-in law. Also, my mother-in-law is less guarded and [more] accepting of our assistance. She is more appreciative and pleasant than in the past.

I have learned to treasure the memories of all the good years instead of mourning the loss of the years we might have had together.

A social worker who worked with individuals and families affected by AD prior to the onset of her mother's AD reports:

Having this personal experience both deepened and added another dimension to my professional life. I don't mean to say that professionals who don't have this experience can't be excellent—there are many. Another positive is the loving, intimate, and spiritual connection it provided both my mother and me. We would not have reached this level in our relationship without her Alzheimer's. It was truly a gift.

LESSONS LEARNED

It is difficult to encapsulate the varied experiences of people who have cared for a loved one with AD. It is even more difficult to explain why people cope poorly or well with a similar set of challenges day after day, year after year. The quality of one's past relationship with the person with AD influences one's coping ability. The amount and frequency of social supports certainly make a difference too. Other personal resources, such as time and money, can also play roles. A vast amount of social research in recent years has looked at a variety of factors that help explain why some people cope poorly and why others cope well caring for a loved one with AD. An interesting finding has emerged: Above all else, how one perceives the situation accounts for much of the difference in whether one copes poorly or well.

Those who see this situation as an ongoing tragedy typically respond to the stressors with depression, anxiety, and a host of other problems. They perceive no positive results from their hard work and they often feel depleted. The deterioration of a loved one's mind is a cause for daily sadness. They see little or nothing good in the present situation and truly suffer through an endless funeral. Despair is an everyday reality and the future looks grim.

On the other hand, those who learn to see a loved one's AD as an opportunity to achieve personal meaning, mission, or purpose are likely to cope well. Their countless acts of devotion, although draining at times, lead them not to despair but to confirmation that each day is worthwhile. They accept the limits imposed by AD yet try to realize the potential in every encounter and act of care. They see problems as challenges that can lead to personal growth. They see with eyes of faith, irrespective of a religious bent, and understand that a broken mind or body is not the ultimate tragedy. They are most concerned with care of the soul— their loved one's and their own.

You cannot give what you do not have. If you cannot be open to the possibilities presented by AD, then seek out help—you will be amazed to find other people who have learned to thrive, not just survive. You can change your attitude and behavior to adapt to this life-changing situation. Human resilience in the face of adversity is a wonder to behold. Your loved one with AD will benefit from your personal struggle and you will eventually grow beyond measure into a better person.

Finally, I wish to end with a call for courage. You have an awesome responsibility to ensure that someone with AD lives life to the fullest, no matter how radically that may differ from his or her past standards. At the same time, you also must make sure that your life is kept in balance in spite of the sacrifices you make every day. Winston Churchill implored the people of Great Britain in the midst of World War II to continue struggling for hope and his message may well apply to you now:

> "Never give in, never give in, never, never, never, never—in nothing, great or small, large or petty—never give in except to convictions of honor and good sense."

. . . .
.
.
.

Advocating for Change

*It is not enough for a great nation
merely to have added new years to
life. Our objective must also be to
add new life to those years.*

John F. Kennedy

I f you are a relative or friend directly involved in providing care
to someone with AD, you are probably spending a lot of time
and energy dealing with it every day. Although the problems
associated with the disease are shared by millions of people, your
focus is probably on the personal or family issues related to the
disease and not on the larger social context. While it may be unrealistic right now for you to be involved in advocating for changes
in public policy that would improve care and lead to better treatments or prevention, you should be aware of the larger issues in
the political arena. The problem of AD is far too big and complex
for any individual or family to solve, and advocates are needed in
the long-running battles over public policy and funding.

Until recently in American society, several generations of
families typically lived fairly close together. Mutual assistance in
caring for the needs of the young and old alike was a clear expectation in extended families. The responsibility of caring for a sick

or disabled relative was likewise often shared among members of the family. For a variety of reasons, families ordinarily do not enjoy such close ties today. The responsibility of caring for the young and old is now shared by fewer family members than ever before in human history. Too often the care of someone with a severe or disabling illness like AD falls on the shoulders of one person. Unfortunately, no individual can successfully meet the long-term needs of someone with AD, and various forms of help, such as that provided by relatives, friends, neighbors, employers, churches, civic organizations, and government programs are needed.

When Hillary Rodham Clinton wrote her book based on the African adage "It takes a village to raise a child," she was criticized for trying to substitute government for the role of individuals. She responded by saying that the task of child rearing is so crucial to society that it needs to be seen as both a personal and collective endeavor. This same argument might well apply to the task of caring for someone with AD. The disease takes a heavy toll on society—everyone pays, either directly or indirectly. And AD presents enormous financial problems as well, costing well over $100 billion annually in the United States alone.[1] Although most costs are borne privately, the costs to government and business are already huge and will continue to grow as the number of people with AD increases in the coming decades.

THE POLITICS OF HEALTH CARE

Any time huge numbers of Americans have been affected by a health problem as significant as AD, there has been a political movement to demand more funding for research and improved care. The public health problems of tuberculosis and polio in past decades led to massive increases in government expenditure to deal with these illnesses. Most recently, significant increases in government allocations devoted to AIDS and breast cancer can be traced directly to grassroots advocacy by people with these diseases, their loved ones, and health-care professionals. The AIDS crisis, in particular, which began in the early 1980s, consolidated the political power of gays and lesbians like no other cause and focused the public's attention like no other health problem had in recent times. The organized efforts of advocates can clearly instill the political will to increase government funding for care, treatment, and prevention of major diseases.

The problem of AD does not yet have a high profile in spite of the staggering human and financial costs. Those with the disease are seldom able to speak for themselves. They cannot mount letter-writing campaigns, march in public demonstrations, or lobby elected officials to express dissatisfaction over the state of funding for care, treatment, and prevention of AD. For the most part, they are older people who are hidden in the shadows and easily ignored by the rest of society. They are considered "over the hill" and hold no political power. Furthermore, their loved ones, directly engaged in caring for them, are too busy to be involved in a demanding political movement.

The Alzheimer's Association, Alzheimer Society, and similar organizations have been remarkably effective in increasing public awareness and raising federal allocations for AD research every year over the past twenty years. However, although the total amount allocated for AD research from U.S. government funds continues to grow each year, research expenditures pale in comparison to other major public health problems. Advocates are needed to raise funds and to pressure elected officials into allocating a much bigger portion of government funds. The Alzheimer's Association is the leading organization in this advocacy effort in the United States. Contact the national office at (312) 335-8700 or at (800) 272-3900 for information about what you can do to join and help. Likewise, contact the Alzheimer Society in Canada at (416) 488-8772 or toll-free from within Canada at (800) 616-8816.

If concern about the health of our elders does not generate public concern about AD, then self-interest should. By the year 2050, as many as fourteen million Americans and more than a hundred million people worldwide will have the disease.[2] Women in particular carry a greater burden than men in relation to AD and the disease should rightfully be championed as a women's health issue. Not only do more women than men have AD, but women also provide a disproportionate amount of care to people with the disease. It does not take a crystal ball to predict what will happen in the decades ahead as more people are affected by this chronic condition. It is as if we are standing at the ocean's shore and can see a hurricane approaching from afar, all the while hoping that science will solve the problem before the storm hits. Wishful thinking and denial will not make the problem go away.

THE ROLE OF GOVERNMENT

Progress is being made to find better treatments and means of prevention for AD. Preventing the disease is the ultimate goal of biomedical research, yet this is still just a dream. Robert Butler, M.D., former director of the National Institute on Aging, has cautioned:

> We remain ill-prepared for the twenty-first century when population aging will become unprecedented.... I regard the baby boomers as a generation at risk. We still devote relatively few resources to understanding the biology of aging. Although we have made progress in understanding the pathogenesis of Alzheimer's disease, we are a long way from a cure.[3]

Despite significant advances over the past two decades, it may take many more decades before dramatic results can be seen.

Scientific efforts need better funding to speed up the rate of progress. An annual budget of $1 billion dollars, contributed by the U.S. government for AD research, would begin to put the disease on a par with cancer, heart disease, and AIDS. Devoting 15 percent of that amount to research into finding better ways of caring for people with the disease and their families would underscore the importance of the psychosocial aspects of the disease.

On the other hand, the fate of millions of people cannot be entrusted entirely to the hard-working scientists aiming to unlock the mysteries of AD. There must also be increased attention given to helping those who are currently coping with the disease who will never taste the fruits of scientific progress. Their quality of life depends more on human compassion and skill than on new medical breakthroughs. What can be done to help individuals and families on a practical level? The following are some ideas:

▶ Family members and others who provide direct care should receive increased tax credits in recognition of their hard work and cost savings to society.

▶ In the United States, Medicare and Medicaid must be redesigned to address long-term-care needs and to pay for a portion of prescription drugs and community-based services like home care and adult day care. Medicare is the primary health insurance of people with AD, but it is outdated in light of the common chronic illnesses affecting the elderly and disabled population. Physicians, nurses, social workers, and other health-care professionals need better reimbursement for their services for the sake of preventing people with AD from being admitted into hospitals and other care facilities.

▶ There should be government incentives at all levels to develop alternatives to nursing-home care, such as home care, assisted-living facilities, and other supportive living arrangements. A comprehensive family support network must be established. In the United States, the National Family Caregiving Support Program is now making a positive difference in the lives of families, but this program needs a big budget boost to $1 billion.

▶ Families need easy access to affordable training, education, and counseling programs to support them in their role as the main providers of care. For example, in order to improve medical care for its nearly 500,000 residents with AD, the state of California funded an education campaign aimed at people with AD, their families, and physicians. Other states should fund similar education campaigns in light of the huge communication gap that exists between consumers and physicians.

▶ Technology must be developed and made available that provides on-line information, services, and connections to families coping with AD. For example, computer-based systems, such as the Comprehensive Health

Enhancement Support System (CHESS), developed by the University of Wisconsin, and California's Link2Care, operated by Family Caregiver Alliance, should be made readily accessible to everyone concerned about AD.

THE ROLE OF THE PRIVATE SECTOR

Government alone cannot solve the range of problems associated with AD. Business already pays a high price for this disease, at least $60 billion annually, according to a survey commissioned by the Alzheimer's Association.[4] Absenteeism and tardiness affect an estimated one-third of employees who care for relatives with AD, and 10 percent quit their jobs each year because of their competing roles at work and at home. In response to such family-related concerns, many employers have developed elder-care assistance programs. These include benefits such as

- unpaid leave beyond the twelve-week leave required by the U.S. Family and Medical Leave Act that also guarantees workers retention of full medical and dental benefits, enabling workers to use their sick leave to care for a disabled relative.

- referral services linking employees to services nationwide, making it possible to arrange care for a relative who lives either locally or far away.

- reimbursement for services paid for a disabled relative, similar to child-care reimbursement.

- flexible spending accounts that allow for pretax income to be set aside and reimbursed upon receipt of services.

- long-term-care insurance packages for employees, spouses, parents, and in-laws.

- counseling for employees and their family members affected by care responsibilities.

Government and business can have powerful effects on the quality of life for individuals and families affected by AD. For example, AmeriCorps, a national service program of the U.S. government that subsidizes volunteers working with nonprofit organizations, could make AD a priority area and focus directly on services to people affected by the disease, whether they live at home or in care facilities. Churches, synagogues, schools, universities, hospitals, social service agencies, and philanthropic organizations can also devote increased resources to the problems associated with AD. The monthly "Alzheimer's Cafes" springing up in Europe illustrate how private organizations can be helpful in bringing together people with AD, their families, volunteers, and professionals for a mix of education, consultation, emotional support, and social interaction. Cooperation is necessary among different parties to create a variety of programs and to enlist volunteers to support individuals and families dealing with the disease in every community.

There have been many ups and downs in the relatively brief history of research into the causes, treatment, and prevention of AD. Success in the end will depend in large part on funding from public and private sources, particularly in the United States. The goal of preventing AD will ultimately be realized when a critical mass of people decides that this is a priority worth funding on a large scale. In the meantime, the goal of improving the quality of life of millions of individuals and families affected by the disease requires increased funding too. The sign that Ronald Reagan kept on his desk in the Oval Office might well be adopted as the motto of everyone working toward these goals: IT CAN BE DONE. This same sense of optimism must fuel the hopes of all who are concerned about this mind-robbing disease, especially those with the disease who can no longer speak for themselves.

Notes

. . . .

Chapter 1: The Need for an Accurate Diagnosis

1. R. C. Peterson et al., "Mild Cognitive Impairment: Clinical Characterization and Outcome," *Archives of Neurology* 56, no. 3 (1999): 303–8.

2. J. C. Morris et al., "Mild Cognitive Impairment Represents Early-Stage Alzheimer's Disease," *Archives of Neurology* 58 (2001): 397–405; D. A. Bennett et al., "Natural History of Mild Cognitive Impairment in Older Persons," *Neurology* 59 (2002): 198–205.

3. B. Kolb and I. Q. Whishaw, *Fundamentals of Human Neuropsychology* (New York: W. H. Freeman, 1990), 4.

4. A. Alzheimer, "Uber eine eigenartige Erkrankung der Hirnrinde," *Allgemeine Zeitschrift für Psychiatrie und Psychisch-Gerichtliche Medizin* 64 (1907): 146–48; A. Alzheimer et al. An English translation of Dr. Alzheimer's "Uber eine eigenartige Erkankung der Hirnrinde" or "A Characteristic Disease of the Cerebral Cortex," *Clinical Anatomy* 8, no. 6 (1995): 429–31.

5. AARP and Administration on Aging, *A Profile of Older Americans 2001* (Washington, DC: AARP, 2001).

6. D. A. Evans et al., "Estimated Prevalence of Alzheimer's Disease in the United States," *Milbank Memorial Fund Quarterly* 68 (1990): 267–89.

7. R. J. Killiany et al., "Use of Structural Magnetic Resonance Imaging to Predict Who Will Get Alzheimer's Disease," *Annals of Neurology* 47, no. 4 (2000): 430–39; R. C. Peterson et al., "Memory and MRI-based Hippocampal Volumes in Aging and AD," *Neurology* 54, no. 3 (2000): 581–7; G. W. Small et al., "In Vivo Brain Imaging of Tangle Burden in Humans," *Jounal of Molecular Neuroscience* 19, no. 3 (2002):323–7.

8. M. F. Folstein, S. E. Folstein, and P. R. McHugh, "Mini-Mental State: A Practical Method for Grading the Cognitive State of Patients for the Clinician," *Journal of Psychiatric Research* 12 (1975): 189–98.

9. G. McKann et al., "Clinical Diagnosis of Alzheimer's Disease: Report of the NINCDS-ADRDA Work Group Under the Auspices of the Department of Health and Human Services Task Force on Alzheimer's Disease," *Neurology* 34 (1984): 939–44; American Psychiatric Association, *The Diagnostic and Statistical Manual of Mental Disorders*, 4th ed. (Washington, DC: American Psychiatric Association, 1994).

10. S. S. Mirra et al., The Consortium to Establish a Registry for Alzheimer's Disease (CERAD), "Standardization of the Neuropathologic Assessment of Alzheimer's Disease," *Neurology* 41 (1991): 479–84; M. F. Mendez et al., "Clinically Diagnosed Alzheimer's Disease: Neuropathologic Findings in 650 Cases," *Alzheimer's Disease and Associated Disorders* 6, no. 35 (1992); J. T. Becker et al., "The Natural History of Alzheimer's Disease: Description of Study Cohort and Accuracy of Diagnosis," *Archives of Neurology* 51 (1994): 585–90.

11. Unless otherwise noted, all quotes are taken from the author's files; identifying details have been altered to protect confidentiality.

12. D. Roland, *Alzheimer's Disease: Communicating With the Patient* (video) (Research Triangle Park, NC: GlaxoWellcome, Inc., 1995).

Chapter 2: Symptoms of the Early Stages of Alzheimer's Disease

1. R. Reagan, "Open Letter to the American Public" (4 November 1994). Available online at: www.reagan.utexas.edu/resource/handout/Alzheime.htm.

2. M. J. Zuckerman, "Bush: Reagan Wasn't Ill as President," *USA Today*, 29 November 1996.

3. E. Morris, *Dutch: A Memoir of Ronald Reagan* (New York: Random House, 1999).

4. "Muskie Amazed by President's Memory Lapses," *Los Angeles Times*, 2 March 1987, sec. 1, p. 1; J. O'Shea and J. Cawley, "Panel Rips Regan, Reagan: President Seen as 'Unaware' in Iran-Contra Deal," *The Chicago Tribune*, 27 February 1987, sec.1, p. 1.

5. A. Davidson, *Alzheimer's, A Love Story: One Year in My Husband's Journey* (Secaucus, NJ: Carol Publishing Group, 1997), 184.

6. K. A. Bayles, "Alzheimer's Disease Symptoms: Prevalence and Order of Symptoms," *The Journal of Applied Gerontology* 10, no. 4 (1991): 419–30.

7. L. Tennis, "Alzheimer's Diary: I Have What!" *The Caregiver* (Winter 1992): 6–13.

8. G. Binetti et al., "Visual and Spatial Perception in the Early Phases of Alzheimer's Disease," *Neuropsychology* 12, no. 1 (1998): 29–33.

9. D. P. Devanand et al., "The Course of Psychopathologic Features in Mild to Moderate Alzheimer's Disease," *Archives of General Psychiatry* 54, no. 3 (1997): 257–63.

10. C. Derousne et al., "Sexual Behavioral Changes in Alzheimer's Disease," *Alzheimer's Disease and Associated Disorders* 10, no. 2 (1996): 86–92; L. K. Wright, "The Impact of Alzheimer's Disease on the Marital Relationship," *The Gerontologist* 21, no. 2 (1991): 224–37; A. M. Zeiss et al., "The Incidence and Correlates of Erectile Problems in Patients with Alzheimer's Disease," *Archives of Sexual Behavior* 19, no. 4 (1991): 325–31.

11. M. Sano et al., "Simple Reaction Time as a Measure of Global Attention in Alzheimer's Disease," *Journal of the International Neuropsychological Society* 1, no. 1 (1995): 56–61; B. R. Ott et al., "Quantitative Assessment of Movement in Alzheimer's Disease," *Journal of Geriatric Psychiatry and Neurology* 8, no. 1 (1995): 71–75.

12. R. I. Mesholam et al., "Olfaction in Neurodegenerative Disease: A Meta-Analysis of Olfactory Functioning in Alzheimer's and Parkinson's Diseases," *Archives of Neurology* 55, no. 1 (1998): 84–90; G. S. Soloman et al., "Olfactory Dysfunction Discriminates Alzheimer's Dementia from Major Depression," *Journal of Neuropsychiatry and Clinical Neuroscience* 10, no. 1 (1998): 64–67.

Chapter 3: Risk Factors for Developing Alzheimer's Disease

1. D. A. Evans et al., "Prevalence of Alzheimer's Disease in a Community Population Higher Than Previously Reported," *Journal of the American Medical Association* 262 (1989): 2251–56.

2. National Institute on Aging, *Progress Report on Alzheimer's Disease 2000* (Bethesda, MD: U.S. Department of Health and Human Services, National Institutes of Health, National Institute on Aging, 2001). Also available on-line at: www.alzheimers.org/pubs/prog00.htm

3. World Health Organization, *World Health Report 2001, Mental Health: New Understanding, New Hope.* Geneva, Switzerland: 2001. Also available on-line at: www.who.int/whr/2001/main/

4. J. C. Breitner et al., "Familial Aggregation in Alzheimer's Disease: Comparison of Risk Among Relatives of Early- and Late-Onset Cases, and Among Male and Female Relatives in Successive Generations," *Neurology* 38 (1988): 207–12.

5. P. St. George-Hyslop et al., "The Genetic Defect Causing Familial Alzheimer's Disease Maps on Chromosome 21," *Science* 235 (1987): 885–90; G. D. Schellenberg et al., "Genetic Linkage Evidence for a Familial Alzheimer's Disease Locus on Chromosome 14," *Science* 258, no. 5082 (1992): 668–71; E. Levy-Lahad et al., "Candidate Gene for the Chromosome 1 Familial Alzheimer's Disease Locus," *Science* 269, no. 5226 (1995): 973–77.

6. S. G. Post and P. J. Whitehouse, *Genetic Testing for Alzheimer's Disease: Ethical and Clinical Issues* (Baltimore, MD: The Johns Hopkins University Press, 1998).

7. E. H. Corder et al., "Gene Dose of Apolipoprotein in E Type 4 Allele and the Risk of Alzheimer's Disease in Late-Onset Families," *Science* 261, no. 5123 (1993): 921–23.

8. D. A. Evans et al., "Apolipoprotein A Epsilon4 and Incidence of Alzheimer's Disease in a Community Population of Older Persons," *Journal of the American Medical Association* 227 (1997): 822–24.

9. A. Myers et al., "Susceptibility Locus for Alzheimer's Disease on Chromosome 10," *Science* 290, no. 5500 (2000): 2304–5; L. Betram et al., "Evidence for Genetic Linkage of Alzheimer's Disease to Chromosome 10q," *Science* 290, no. 5500. (2000): 2302–3.

10. The Ronald and Nancy Reagan Research Institute of the Alzheimer's Association and the National Institute on Aging Working Group. Consensus Report of the Working Group, "Molecular and Biochemical Markers of Alzheimer's Disease," *Neurobiology of Aging* 19, no. 2 (1998): 109–16; R. Mayeux et al., for the Alzheimer's Disease Centers Consortium on Apolipoprotein E and Alzheimer's Disease, "Utility of the Apolipoprotein E Genotype in the Diagnosis of Alzheimer's Disease," *New England Journal of Medicine* 338, no. 8 (1998): 506–11.

11. K. E. Wisniewski, H. M. Wisniewski, and G. Y. Wen, "Occurrence of Neuropathological Changes and Dementia of Alzheimer's Disease in Down's Syndrome," *Annals of Neurology* 17 (1985): 278–82.

12. F. E. Visser et al., "Prospective Study of the Prevalence of Alzheimer-Type Dementia in Institutionalized Individuals with Down's Syndrome," *American Journal of Mental Retardation* 101 (1997): 400–12.

13. A. Heyman et al., "Alzheimer's Disease: A Study of Epidemiological Aspects," *Annals of Neurology* 15 (1984): 335–41; R. Mayeux et al., "Genetic Susceptibility and Head Injury as Risk Factors for Alzheimer's Disease Among Community-Dwelling Persons and Their First-Degree Relatives," *Annals of Neurology* 33 (1993): 494–501; P. N. Nemetz et al., "Traumatic Head Injury and Time to Onset of Alzheimer's Disease: A Population Study," *American Journal of Epidemiology* 149 (1999): 32–40.

14. P. W. Schofield et al., "Alzheimer's Disease After Remote Head Injury," *Journal of Neurology, Neurosurgery and Psychiatry* 62 (1997): 119–24; Z. Guo et al., "Head Injury and the Risk of AD in the MIRAGE Study," *Neurology* 54, no. 6 (2000): 1316–23.

15. D. A. Evans et al., "Education and Other Measures of Socioeconomic Status and Risk of Incident Alzheimer's Disease in a Defined Population of Older Persons," *Archives of Neurology* 54, no. 11 (1997): 1399–1405; Y. Stern et al., "Influence of Education and Occupation on the Incidence of Alzheimer's Disease, *Journal of the American Medical Association* 271, no. 13 (1994): 1004–10; L. White et al, "Association of Education with Incidence of Cognitive Impairment in Three Established Populations for Epidemiologic Studies of the Elderly, *Journal of Clinical Epidemiology* 47 (1994): 363–70.

16. H. Payami et al., "Increased Risk of Familial Late-Onset Alzheimer's Disease in Women," *Neurology* 46 (1996): 126–29; L. J. Launer et al., "Rates and Risk Factors for Dementia and Alzheimer's Disease: Results from the EURODEM Pooled Analyses," *Neurology* 52 (1999): 78–84; L. Letenneur et al., "Are Sex and Educational Level Independent Predictors of Dementia and Alzheimer's Disease? Incidence Data from the PAQUID Project," *Journal of Neurology, Neurosurgery and Psychiatry* 66 (1999): 177–83.

17. D. A. Snowden et al., "Brain Infarction and the Clinical Expression of Alzheimer's Disease: The Nun Study," *Journal of the American Medical Association* 277, no. 10 (1997): 813–17.

18. R. Mayeux et al., "An Estimated Prevalence of Dementia in Parkinson's Disease," *Archives of Neurology* 45 (1988): 260–62; E. Mohr, T. Mendis, and J. D. Grimes, "Late Cognitive Changes in Parkinson's Disease with an Emphasis on Dementia," in *Behavioral Neurology of Movement Disorders*, W. J. Weiner and A. E. Lang, eds. (New York: Raven Press, 1995), 97–113.

19. A. Heyman et al., "Estimated Prevalence of Dementia Among Elderly Black and White Community Residents," *Archives of Neurology* 48 (1991): 594–98.

20. M. X. Tang et al., "The APOE-E4 Allele and the Risk of Alzheimer's Disease Among African-Americans, Whites and Hispanics," *Journal of the American Medical Association* 279, no. 10 (1998): 751–55.

21. L. White et al., "Prevalence of Dementia in Older Japanese-American Men in Hawaii," *Journal of the American Medical Association* 276, no. 12 (1996): 955–60.

22. R. A. Armstrong, S. J. Winsper, and J. A. Blair, "Aluminum and Alzheimer's Disease: Review of Possible Pathogenic Mechanisms," *Dementia* 7, no 1 (1996): 1–9; J. Savory et al., "Can the Controversy of the Role of Aluminum in Alzheimer's Disease be Resolved?" *Journal of Toxicity and Environmental Health* 48, no. 6 (1996): 615–35.

23. W. R. Markesbury, "Trace Elements in Alzheimer's Disease," in *Alzheimer's Disease: Cause(s), Diagnosis, Treatment, and Care*, Z. S. Khachaturian and T. S. Radebaugh, eds. (Boca Raton, FL: CRC Press, 1996), 233–36; S. R. Saxe et al., "Alzheimer's Disease, Dental Amalgam and Mercury," *Journal of the American Dental Association* 130 (1999): 191–99.

24. W. A. Kukall et al., "Solvent Exposure as a Risk Factor for Alzheimer's Disease: A Case-Control Study," *American Journal of Epidemiology* 141, no. 11 (1995): 1059–71.

25. Canadian Study of Health and Aging Investigators, "The Canadian Study of Health and Aging: Risk Factors for Alzheimer's Disease in Canada," *Neurology* 40 (1994): 1492–95.

26. E. Sobel et al., "Elevated Risk of Alzheimer's Disease Among Workers with Likely Electromagnetic Field Exposure," *Neurology* 47, no. 6 (1996): 1477–81; M. Feychting et al., "Dementia and Occupational Exposure to Magnetic Fields," *Scandinavian Journal of Work and Environmental Health* 24, no 1 (1998): 46–53.

27. A. Ott et al., "Smoking and the Risk of Dementia and Alzheimer's Disease in a Population-Based Cohort Study: The Rotterdam Study," *Lancet* 351, no. 9119 (1998): 1840–43.

28. C. Merchant et al., "The Influence of Smoking on the Risk of Alzheimer's Disease," *Neurology* 52, no. 7 (1999): 1408–12; A. Ott et al., for the EURODEM Incidence Research Group, "Smoking Is a Risk Factor for Cognitive Decline in Non-Demented Elderly: The

EURODEM Studies," *Neurology* 50, no. 4 Suppl. (1998): Presentation at the Fiftieth Annual Meeting of the American Academy of Neurology, Minneapolis, MN: 29 April 1998.

29. A. B. Graves et al., "Alcohol and Tobacco Consumption as Risk Factors for Alzheimer's Disease: A Collaborative Re-analysis of Case-Control Studies," *International Journal of Epidemiology* 20, no. 2 Suppl. (1991): S48–57; L. Lettenneur et al., "Tobacco Consumption and Cognitive Impairment in Elderly People: A Population-Based Study," *Annals of Epidemiology* 4, no. 6 (1994): 449–54.

30. P. A. Newhouse, A. Potter, and E. D. Levin, "Nicotinic System Involvement in Alzheimer's and Parkinson's Disease: Implications for Therapeutics," *Drugs and Aging* 11, no. 3 (1997): 206–28.

31. S. Kalmijn et al., "Polyunsaturated Fatty Foods, Antioxidants, and Cognitive Function in the Very Old," *American Journal of Epidemiology* 145 (1994): 33–41; J. A. Luchinger et al., "Caloric Intake and Alzheimer's Disease," *Archives of Neurology* 59, no. 8 (2002): 1258–63.

32. R. Clarke et al., "Folate, Vitamin B 12, and Serum Total Homocysteine Levels in Confirmed Alzheimer's Disease," *Archives of Neurology* 55 (1998): 1449–55; S. Seshadri et al., "Plasma Homocysteine as a Risk Factor for Alzheimer's Disease," *The New England Journal of Medicine* 46, no 7 (2002): 476–83.

33. A. L. Smith et al., "The Protective Effects of Life-Long, Regular Physical Exercise on the Development of Alzheimer's Disease," *Neurology* 50, no. 4 Suppl. (1998): Presentation at the Fiftieth Annual Meeting of the American Academy of Neurology, Minneapolis, MN: 29 April 1998; C. W. Cotman and N. C. Berchtold, "Exercise: A Behavioral Intervention to Enhance Brain Health and Plasticity," *Trends in Neurosciences* 25 (2002): 6; J. Lindsay et al., "Risk Factors for Alzheimer's Disease: A Prospective Analysis from the Canadian Study of Health and Aging," *American Journal of Epidemiology* 156, no 5 (2002): 445–53.

34. K. Yaffe et al., "Serum Lipoprotein Levels, Statin Use, and Cognitive Function in Older Women," *Archives of Neurology* 59, no. 3 (2002): 378–84; E. van Exel et al., "Association between High-Density Lipoprotein and Cognitive Impairment in the Oldest Old," *Annals of Neurology* 51, no. 5 (2002): 716–21; L. J. Launer et al., "Cholesterol and Neuropathic Markers of AD: A Population-Based Autopsy Study," *Neurology* 57, no. 8 (2001): 1447–52.

35. A. F. Jorm et al., "Psychiatric History and Related Exposures as Risk Factors for Alzheimer's Disease," *International Journal of Epidemiology* 20, Suppl. 2 (1991): S43–47.

36. R. Yehuda et al., "Dose-Response Changes in Plasma Cortisol and Lymphocyte Glucocorticoid Receptors Following Dexamethasone Administration in Combat Veterans With and Without Posttraumatic Stress Disorder," *Archives of General Psychiatry* 52, no. 7 (1995): 583–93; R. Yehuda et al., "Learning and Memory in Combat Veterans with Posttraumatic Stress Disorder," *American Journal of Psychiatry* 152, no. 1 (1995): 137–39.

37. C. E. Speck et al., "History of Depression as a Risk Factor for Alzheimer's Disease, *Epidemiology* 6, no. 4 (1995): 366–69; J. L. Wetherell et al., "History of Depression and Other Psychiatric Illness as Risk Factors for Alzheimer's Disease in a Twin Sample," *Alzheimer's Disease and Associated Disorders* 13, no. 1 (1999): 47–52; R. S. Wilson et al., "Depressive Symptoms, Cognitive Decline, and Risk of AD in Older Persons," *Neurology* 59 (2002): 364–370.

38. National Institutes of Health, "Diagnosis and Treatment of Depression in Late Life," *NIH Consensus Statement* 9, no. 3 (1991): 1–27.

39. A. S. Henderson, "Co-occurrence of Affective and Cognitive Symptoms: The Epidemiological Evidence," *Dementia* 1 (1990): 119–23; R. Migliorelli et al., "Prevalence and Correlates of Dysthmia and Major Depression Among Patients with Alzheimer's Disease," *American Journal of Psychiatry* 152 (1995): 37–44; Y. Forsell and B. Wingblad, "Major Depression in a Population of Demented and Nondemented Older People: Prevalence and Correlates," *Journal of the American Geriatrics Society* 46 (1998): 27–30.

40. J. S. Kennedy and P. Whitehouse, "Alzheimer's Disease," in *Clinical Geriatric Neurology*, L. Barclay, ed. (Malvern, PA: Lea and Febinger, 1993), 76–89.

41. G. S. Alexopoulos et al., eds., *The Expert Consensus Guideline Series: Treatment of Agitation in Older Persons with Dementia*. A Special Report of Postgraduate Medicine, April 1998, 68. Minneapolis, MN: McGraw-Hill Healthcare Information Programs. Also available online at www.psychguides.com/gl-treatment_of_agitation_in_dementia.html.

Chapter 4: Progress in Treatment and Prevention of Alzheimer's Disease

1. N. Qizilbash et al., "Cholinesterase Inhibition for Alzheimer's Disease: A Meta-analysis of the Tacrine Trials," *Journal of the American Medical Association* 280, no. 20 (1998): 1777–82; S. L. Rogers et al., "A 24-Week, Double-Blind, Placebo-Controlled Trial of Donepezil in Patients with Alzheimer's Disease," *Neurology* 50 (1998): 136–45; M. W. Jann, "Rivastigmine: A New Generation Cholinesterase Inhibitor for the Treatment of Alzheimer's Disease," *Pharmacotherapy* 20 (2000): 1–12; P. N. Tariot et al., "A 5-Month, Randomized, Placebo-Controlled Trail of Galantamine in AD. USA-10 Study Group." *Neurology* 54, no. 12 (2000): 2269–76.

2. R. S. Doody et al., "Open-Label, Multicenter, Phase 3 Extension Study of the Safety and Efficacy of Donepezil in Patients with Alzheimer's Disease," *Archives of Neurology* 58, no. 3 (2001): 427–33.

3. R. Bullock and C. Connolly, "Switching Cholinesterase Inhibitor Therapy in Alzheimer's Disease—Donepezil to Rivastigmine, Is It Worth It?" *International Journal of Geriatric Psychiatry* 17 (2002): 288–89.

4. J. L. Cummings et al., "Alzheimer's Disease: Etiologies, Pathophysiology, Cognitive Reserve, and Treatment Opportunities," *Neurology* 51, Suppl. 1 (1998): S2–17; P. N. Tariot, L. Schneider, and A. P. Porteinsson, "Treating Alzheimer's Disease: Pharmacologic Options Now and in the Near Future," *Postgraduate Medicine* 101, no. 6 (1997): 73–90.

5. P. L. McGeer, M. Schulzer, and E. G. McGeer, "Arthritis and Anti-Inflammatory Agents as Possible Protective Factors for Alzheimer's Disease: A Review of 17 Epidemiologic Studies," *Neurology* 47 (1996): 425–32; W. F. Stewart et al., "Risk of Alzheimer's Disease and Duration of NSAID Use," *Neurology* 48 (1997): 626–32; J. B. Rich et al., "Nonsteroidal Anti-inflammatory Drugs in Alzheimer's Disease," *Neurology* 46 (1995): 626–32.

6. P. Aisen et al., "Results of a Multicenter Trial of Rofocoxeib and Naproxen in Alzheimer's Disease," Paper presentation at 8th International Conference on Alzheimer's Disease and Related Disorders. Stockholm, Sweden: 24 July 2002.

7. R. C. Green et al., "Statin Use is Associated with Reduced Risk of Alzheimer's Disease," *Neurology* 58 (2002) A81; B. Wolozin et al., "Decreased Prevalence of Alzheimer Disease Associated with 3-hydroxy-3-methyglutaryl coenzyme A Reductase Inhibitors," *Archives of Neurology* 57, no. 10 (2000): 1439–43.

8. R. Mulnard et al., "Estrogen Replacement Therapy Not Effective for Treatment of Mild Alzheimer's Disease: A Randomized Controlled Trial," *Journal of the American Medical Association* 238, no. 8 (2000): 1007–1015; V. H. Henderson et al., "Estrogen for Alzheimer's Disease in Women: Randomized, Double-blind, Placebo-controlled Trial," *Neurology* 54, no. 2 (2000): 295–301; B. Cholerton et al., "Estrogen and Alzheimer's Disease: The Story So Far," *Drugs & Aging* 19, no. 6 (2002) 405–427.

9. Writing Group for the Women's Health Initiative Investigators, "Risks and Benefits of Estrogen Plus Progestin in Healthy Menopausal Women," *Journal of the American Medical Association* 288, no. 3 (2002): 321–333.

10. S. S. Pitchumoni and P. M. Doraiswamy, "Current Status of Antioxidant Therapy for Alzheimer's Disease," *Journal of the American Geriatrics Society* 46 (1998): 1566–72.

11. M. Sano et al., for the Members of the Alzheimer's Disease Cooperative Study, "A Controlled Trial of Selegiline, Alpha-Tocopherol, or Both as Treatment for Alzheimer's Disease," *The New England Journal of Medicine* 336 (1997): 1216–22.

12. M. C. Morris et al., "Dietary Intake of Antioxidant Nutrients and the Risk of Incident Alzheimer's Disease," *Journal of the American Medical Association* 287, no. 24 (2002): 3230–37; M. J. Englehart et al., "Dietary Intake and Risk of Alzheimer's Disease," *Journal of the American Medical Association* 287, no. 24 (2002): 3223–29.

13. P. L. LeBars et al., "A Placebo-Controlled, Double-Blind Randomized Trial of an Extract of Gingko Biloba for Dementia," *Journal of the American Medical Association* 278, no. 16 (1997): 1327–32.

14. B. S. Oken, D. M. Storzbach, and J. A. Kaye, "The Efficacy of Gingko Biloba on Cognitive Function in Alzheimer's Disease," *Archives of Neurology* 55 (1998): 1409–15.

15. D. H. Cheng, H. Ren, and X. C. Tang, "Huperzine A: A Novel Promising Acetylcholinesterase Inhibitor," *Neuroreport* 8, no. 1 (1996): 97–101; A. A. Skolnick, "Old Chinese Herbal Medicine Used for Fever Yields Possible New Alzheimer's Disease Therapy," *Journal of the American Medical Association* 277, no. 10 (1997): 776.

16. S. Borman, "End Run Around the FDA?" *Chemical and Engineering News* (June 1998): 45–46.

17. G. Kempermann, H. G. Kuhn, and F. H. Gage, "More Hippocampal Neurons in Adult Mice Living in an Enriched Environment," *Nature*

386, no. 6624 (1997): 493–95; M. C. Diamond and J. Hopson, *Magic Trees of the Mind* (New York: Dutton, 1998).

18. C. Fabrigoule et al., "Social and Leisure Activities and Risk of Dementia: A Prospective Longitudinal Study," *Journal of the American Geriatrics Society* 43 (1995): 485–90; R. S. Wilson et al., "Participation in Cognitively Stimulating Activities and Risk of Incident Alzheimer's Disease," *Journal of the American Medical Association* 287 (2002): 742–48.

19. Quoted in W. B. Bean, *Sir William Osler: Aphorisms from his Bedside Teachings and Writings* (Springfield, IL: Charles C. Thomas, 1961), 77.

Chapter 5: What Is It Like to Have Alzheimer's Disease?

1. C. Henderson et al., *Partial View: An Alzheimer's Journal* (Dallas, TX: Southern Methodist University Press, 1998); R. Davis, *My Journey into Alzheimer's Disease* (Wheaton, IL: Tyndale House Publishers, 1989); L. Rose, *Show Me the Way to Go Home* (Forest Knolls, CA: Elder Books, 1996); D. F. McGowin, *Living in the Labyrinth: A Personal Journey Through the Maze of Alzheimer's* (New York: Delacorte Press, 1993); C. Boden, *Who Will I Be When I Die?* (East Melbourne, Australia: HarperCollins Religious, 1998); T. M. Raushi, *A View from Within: Living with Early Onset Alzheimer's* (Albany, NY: Northeastern Chapter of the Alzheimer's Association, 2001).

2. I. Gatz, ed., *Early Alzheimer's: A Forum for Early Stage Dementia Care* (Santa Barbara, CA: Santa Barbara Alzheimer's Association); L. Snyder, ed., *Perspectives: A Newsletter for Individuals Diagnosed with Alzheimer's Disease* (La Jolla, CA).

3. Henderson, *Partial View*, 36.

4. Henderson, *Partial View*, 55.

5. Davis, *My Journey into Alzheimer's Disease*, 100.

6. Rose, *Show Me the Way to Go Home*, 35.

7. Rose, *Show Me the Way to Go Home*, 35.

8. McGowin, *Living in the Labyrinth*, 80.

9. Boden, *Who Will I Be When I Die?*, 53.

10. Davis, *My Journey into Alzheimer's Disease*, 107.

11. McGowin, *Living in the Labyrinth*, 103.

12. Henderson, *Partial View*, 36.

13. Davis, *My Journey into Alzheimer's Disease,* 119.

14. Boden, *Who Will I Be When I Die?,* 49.

15. Rose, *Show Me the Way to Go Home,* 126.

16. McGowin, *Living in the Labyrinth,* 87.

17. Raushi, *A View from Within,* 119.

18. R. Reagan, "Open Letter to the American Public," (4 November 1994). Available online at: www.reagan.utexas.edu/resource/handout/Alzheime.htm.

19. J. LaBelle, "Not to Twilight, But to Midnight," *A Helping Hand* newsletter (Los Angeles: Alzheimer's Association), 9.

20. S. G. Post, *The Moral Challenge of Alzheimer's Disease* (Baltimore, MD: The Johns Hopkins University Press, 1995), 15.

21. Henderson, *Partial View,* 14.

22. C. Heston, "Open Letter to Friends, Colleagues and Fans," (9 August 2002). Available online at: www.online-shrine.com/heston-alzheimers_text.html or www.cnn.com/2002/SHOWBIZ/News/08/09/heston.statement/index.html.

23. D. Baron, "Alzheimer's Disease: Living with It," *Chicago Sun-Times,* 2 November 1992, 3A, 15.

24. G. Muriel, *I Am Not My Own Person Anymore* video (St. Louis, MO: Washington University Division of Geriatric Psychiatry, 1988).

25. A. Fine, "Coping Mechanisms that Work," *Issues in Focus* newsletter (Cleveland, OH: Cleveland Area Alzheimer's Association, 1997), 8–11.

26. L. Snyder and R. Yale, "Accepting Help: When, What Kind, and Who From?" *Perspectives: A Newsletter for Individuals Diagnosed with Alzheimer's Disease* 2, no. 1 (1996): 1–2.

27. J. W. Anthony, *Ask Dr. Know* newsletter (Cambridge, MA: Eastern Massachusetts Alzheimer's Association, 1997).

28. J. W. Anthony, "Ideas About Alzheimer's," *Perspectives: A Newsletter for Individuals Diagnosed with Alzheimer's Disease* 3, no. 3 (1998): 1–3.

29. R. Migliorelli et al., "Anosognosia in Alzheimer's Disease: A Study of Associated Factors," *Journal of Neuropsychiatry and Clinical Neurosciences* 7 (1995): 338–44.

30. Cleveland Area Alzheimer's Association, *Issues in Focus* newsletter (Cleveland, OH: Cleveland Area Alzheimer's Association, 1994).

31. K. Maurer, S. Volk, and H. Gerbaldo, "Auguste D. and Alzheimer's Disease," *Lancet* 349 (1997): 1546–49.

32. T. Kitwood and K. Bredin, *Person to Person: A Guide to the Care of Those with Failing Mental Powers* (Loughton, England: Gale Centre Publications, 1992); T. Kitwood, *Dementia Reconsidered: The Person Comes First* (Birmingham, England: Open University Press, 1997).

33. Henderson, *Partial View*, 48.

34. Boden, *Who Will I Be When I Die?*, 145.

Chapter 6: How Relationships, Roles, and Responsibilities Change

1. C. M. Clark, *Caring About Howard: Alzheimer's Disease as a Shared Journey* video (Durham, NC: Educational Media Services in association with Lisa Gwyther, Duke University Medical Center, 1997).

2. W. Lustbader, *Counting on Kindness: The Dilemmas of Dependency* (New York: The Free Press, 1992), 79.

3. J. Baron, "Alzheimer's Disease: Living with It," *Chicago Sun-Times*, 2 November 1992, 3A, 15.

4. D. Tilleli, "Reflections." *Perspectives: A Newsletter for Individuals Diagnosed with Alzheimer's Disease* 2, no. 2 (1997): 1–2.

5. L. K. Wright, *Alzheimer's Disease and Marriage* (Newbury Park, CA: Sage Publications, 1993); E. L Ballard and C. Poer, *Sexuality and Alzheimer's Disease* (Durham, NC: Duke University Medical Center, Joseph and Kathleen Bryan Alzheimer's Disease Research Center, 1993); D. R. Kuhn, "The Changing Face of Sexual Intimacy in Alzheimer's Disease," *The American Journal of Alzheimer's Care and Research* 9, no. 5 (1994): 7–14.

6. M. L'Engle, *The Summer of the Great-Grandmother* (New York: Farrar, Strauss & Giroux, 1974), 187.

7. Educational Media Services and L. P. Gwyther, *From Here to Hope: The Stages of Alzheimer's Disease* video (Durham, NC: Duke University Medical Center, 1998).

8. Alzheimer's Association, *Alzheimer's Disease: Inside Looking Out* video (Cleveland, OH: Cleveland Area Chapter, 1995).

9. C. Boden, *Who Will I Be When I Die?* (East Melbourne, Australia: HarperCollins Religious, 1998), 58.

10. D. D. Gray, *I Want To Remember: A Son's Reflection on His Mother's Alzheimer's Journey* (Wellesley, MA: Roundtable Press, 1993).

Chapter 7: Making Practical Decisions

1. M. Rizzo et al., "Simulated Car Crashes at Intersection in Drivers with Alzheimer's Disease," *Alzheimer's Disease and Associated Disorders* 15, (2001): 10–20; L. A. Hunt et al., "Environmental Cueing May Affect Performance on a Road Test for Drivers with Dementia of the Alzheimer Type," *Alzheimer's Disease and Associated Disorders* 11, Suppl. 1 (1997): 13–16; J. M. Duchek et al., "The Role of Selective Attention in Driving and Dementia of the Alzheimer Type," *Alzheimer's Disease and Associated Disorders* 11, Suppl. 1 (1997): 48–56.

2. E. Petrucelli, "Medical Advisory Board Reporting Laws and Medical Licensing Standards," *Proceedings of the Conference on Driver Competency Assessment.* San Diego, CA: California Department of Motor Vehicles, National Research Council, 24–26 October 1990.

3. D. B. Reuben and P. St. George, "Driving and Dementia: California's Approach to a Medical and Policy Dilemma," *Western Journal of Medicine* 164, no. 2 (1996): 111–21.

4. M. Rizzo et al., "Simulated Car Crashes and Crash Predictors in Drivers with Alzheimer's Disease," *Archives of Neurology* 54, no. 5 (1997): 545–51; L. A. Hunt et al., "Reliability of the Washington University Road Test: A Performance-Based Assessment for Drivers with Dementia of the Alzheimer's Type," *Archives of Neurology* 54, no. 6 (1997): 707–12.

5. D. B. Carr et al., "Differentiating Drivers with Dementia of the Alzheimer Type from Healthy Older Persons with a Traffic Sign Naming Test," *Journals of Gerontology: Biological Sciences & Medical Sciences* 53, no. 2 (1998): M135–39.

6. D. K. Helling et al., "Medication Use Characteristics in the Elderly: The Iowa 65 Rural Health Study," *Journal of the American Geriatrics Society* 35 (1987): 4–12.

7. C. Salzman, "Medication Compliance in the Elderly," *Journal of Clinical Psychiatry* 56, Suppl. 1 (1995): 18–22.

8. L. Nerenberg, *Financial Abuse of the Elderly* (Washington, DC: National Center on Elder Abuse, 1996).

9. C. Tom, "Model Advance Directive Combats Financial Abuse," *Aging Today* 20, no. 1 (1999): 10.

10. P. A. Webber, P. Fox, and D. Burnette, "Living Alone with Alzheimer's Disease: Effects on Health and Social Service Utilization Patterns," *Gerontologist* 34, no. 8 (1994): 386–94.

11. Alzheimer's Association, *Alzheimer's Disease: Inside Looking Out* video (Cleveland, OH: Cleveland Area Chapter, 1995).

12. B. B. Murphy, *He Used to Be Somebody: A Journey into Alzheimer's Disease Through the Eyes of a Caregiver* (Boulder, CO: Gibbs Associates, 1995), 311.

Chapter 8: Improving Communication

1. T. Kitwood, *Dementia Reconsidered: The Person Comes First* (Buckingham, England: Open University Press, 1997), 57.

2. D. Barlow, "A Communication Barrier," *Perspectives: A Newsletter for Individuals Diagnosed with Alzheimer's Disease* 3, no. 2 (1998): 6.

3. R. Davis, *My Journey into Alzheimer's Disease* (Wheaton, IL: Tyndale House Publishers, 1989) 85–86.

4. T. Raushi, *A View From Within: Living with Early Onset Alzheimer's* (Albany, NY: Northeastern Chapter of the Alzheimer's Association, 2001), 26.

5. C. Boden, *Who Will I be When I Die?* (East Melbourne, Australia: HarperCollins Religious, 1998), 90.

6. Davis, *My Journey into Alzheimer's Disease*, 88.

7. Boden, *Who Will I Be When I Die?*, 71.

8. P. Davis, *Angels Don't Die: My Father's Gift of Faith* (New York: HarperCollins Publishers, 1995), 36.

9. D. Hoffman, *Complaints of a Dutiful Daughter* video (New York: Women Make Movies, 1995).

10. J. Bow, "Remembering My Husband's Changing Needs," *Rush Alzheimer's Disease Center News* (Winter 1999): 6.

11. A. Davidson, *Alzheimer's, A Love Story: One Year in My Husband's Journey* (Secaucus, NJ: Carol Publishing Group, 1997), 193.

Chapter 9: Helping a Person with AD Plan for the Future

1. Alzheimer's Association, "Taxes and Alzheimer's Disease," Washington, D.C: Alzheimer's Association, Public Policy Office, 1999. (See Print and Video Resources for further information.)

2. A. Haar, "President Clinton Proposes Tax Credits for Long-Term Care," *Provider* (2), no. 9 (1999): 5.

3. J. Vanden Bosch, *A Thousand Tomorrows: Intimacy, Sexuality and Alzheimer's* video (Chicago: Terra Nova Films, 1995).

Chapter 10: Keeping a Person with AD Active and Healthy

1. J. Zgola, "Programming," in *Key Elements of Dementia Care,* Alzheimer's Association, ed. (Chicago: Alzheimer's Association, 1997).

2. C. Boden, *Who Will I Be When I Die?* (East Melbourne, Australia: HarperCollins Religious, 1998), 81.

3. R. N. Davis, P. J. Massman, R. S. Doody, "Cognitive Intervention in Alzheimer's Disease: A Randomized Placebo-Controlled Study," *Alzheimer's Disease and Related Disorders* 15, no. 1 (2001): 1–9.

4. M. S. Bourgeois, *Conversing with Memory-Impaired Individuals Using Memory Aids* (Gaylord, MI: Northern Speech Services, 1992).

5. M. E. Nelson and S. Wernick, *Strong Women Stay Young,* revised edition (New York: Bantam Doubleday Dell Publishing, 2001).

6. University of Michigan, *SMILE Program* (Ann Arbor, MI: School of Public Health, 1994).

7. C. Torkelson, *Get Fit While You Sit: Easy Workouts from Your Chair* (Alameda, CA: Hunter House Publishers Inc., 1999).

8. W. H. Thomas, *Life Worth Living: How Someone You Love Can Still Enjoy Life in a Nursing Home* (Acton, ME: VanderWyk and Burnham, 1996).

Chapter 11: Self-Renewal for Family and Friends

1. R. Schulz and G. M. Williamson, "Health Effects of Caregiving," in *Stress Effects on Family Caregivers of Alzheimer's Patients,* E. Light, G. Neiderehe, and B. Lebowitz, eds. (New York: Springer, 1994); R. Shulz et al., "Psychiatric and Physical Morbidity Effects of Dementia Caregiving: Prevalence, Correlates, and Causes," *The Gerontologist* 35 (1995): 771–91; P. P. Vitaliano et al., "Research on Physiological and Physical Concomitants of Caregiving: Where Do We Go from Here?" *Annals of Behavioral Medicine* 19, no. 2 (1997): 117–23; S. H. Croog et al., "Vulnerability of Husband and Wife Caregivers of Alzheimer Disease Patients to Caregiving Stressors," *Alzheimer Disease and Associated Disorders* 15, no. 4 (2001): 201–10.

2. Alzheimer's Association, *Alzheimer's Disease Caregiver's Survey* (Chicago: Alzheimer's Association, 1996), 3.

3. S. Glick, "Watching Over Leonard," *North Shore Magazine* 32, no. 5 (1999): 56.

4. United States Department of Agriculture, *The Food Guide Pyramid,* Publication HG-252 (Washington, D.C.: U.S. Government Printing Office, 1996); United States Department of Agriculture, *1995 Dietary Guidelines for Americans,* Publication HG-232 (Washington, D.C.: U.S. Government Printing Office, 1995).

5. R. M. Russell, "Nutrition and Health for Older Americans: New Views on the RDAs for Older Adults," *Journal of the American Dietetic Association* 97, no.5 (1997): 515–18; K. Eddy, "Aging Appetites," *Chicago Tribune,* 14 April 1999, Sec. 7, 3.

6. D. Kuhn, "Relieving Stress Through Regular Exercise," *Rush Alzheimer's Disease Center News* (Spring 1994): 8.

7. Kuhn, "Relieving Stress."

8. E. Kübler-Ross, *On Death and Dying* (New York: Macmillan, 1969).

9. W. Ewing, *Tears in God's Bottle: Reflections on Alzheimer's Caregiving* (Tucson, AZ: WhiteStone Circle Press, 1999), 106.

10. S. Fish, *Alzheimer's: Caring for Your Loved One, Caring for Yourself* (Batavia, IL: Lion Publishing Company, 1990), 171.

11. L. Rose, *Show Me the Way to Go Home* (Forest Knolls, CA: Elder Books, 1996), 139.

12. J. Tucker, "How to Change Surviving into Thriving," *Rush Alzheimer's Disease Center News* (Spring 1995): 4.

13. G. Sheehy, *Pathfinders* (New York: Morrow, 1981).

Chapter 12: Obtaining the Help You May Need

1. D. Kuhn, "The Normative Crises of Families Confronting Dementia," *Families in Society: The Journal of Contemporary Human Services* 71, no. 8 (1990): 451–60.

Chapter 13: Voices of Experience

1. W. E. Haley, J. M. Clair, K. Saulsberry, "Family Caregiver Satisfaction With Medical Care of Their Demented Relatives," *Gerontologist* 32, no. 2 (1992): 219–26; S. Holyrod, Q. Turnbull, A. M. Wolf, "What Are Patients and Families Told About Their Diagnosis of Dementia?" *International Journal of Geriatric Psychiatry* 17, no. 3 (2002): 218–21; R. H. Fortinsky, "Health Care Triads and Dementia Care: Integrative

Framework and Future Directions," *Aging and Mental Health* 5 Suppl. 1, no. 2 (2002): 35–48.

2. Roper Starch Worldwide, Inc., *Alzheimer's Disease Study: Communications Gaps Between Physicians and Caregivers* (Chicago: Alzheimer's Association, 2001).

Epilogue: Advocating for Change

1. D. P. Rice et al., "The Economic Burden of Alzheimer's Disease Care," *Health Affairs* 12, no. 2 (1993): 164–76; R. L. Ernst and J. W. Hay, "The U.S. Economic and Social Costs of Alzheimer's Disease Revisited," *American Journal of Public Health* 84 (1994): 1261–64.

2. R. Katzman and P. J. Fox, "The World-Wide Impact of Dementia: Projections of Prevalence and Costs," *Proceedings of Advances in Alzheimer's Disease: Normal Aging, Early Detection and Management of Profound Dementia,* University of California, San Diego, Alzheimer's Disease Research Center Conference, 13–14 May 1999: 11–29.

3. R. J. Hodes, V. Cahan, M. Pruzan, "The National Institute on Aging at Its Twentieth Anniversary: Achievements and Promise of Research on Aging," *Journal of the American Geriatrics Society* 44, no. 2 (1996): 204–6.

4. R. Koppel, *Alzheimer's Disease: The Costs to U.S. Businesses in 2002* (Chicago: Alzheimer's Association, 2002).

Resources

Alzheimer's Disease Centers in the United States Funded Through the National Institute on Aging

These federally funded centers conduct research, offer educational programs about AD for professionals and families, and operate memory disorder clinics. They can refer you to other clinics and services if you do not live near any of them. Also, the National Institute on Aging funds a consortium of research centers, devoted to clinical drug trials, known as the Alzheimer's Disease Cooperative Study. You can contact this consortium at 8950 Villa La Jolla Dr., Ste. 2200, La Jolla, CA 92037; (858) 622-5880; http://antimony.ucsd.edu

In addition to the following centers, several states such as Florida, California, and Illinois fund memory disorder clinics, so check with the Department of Public Health to see if your state has such facilities. Your local chapter of the Alzheimer's Association or Alzheimer Society will also be able to direct you to other AD programs at academic medical centers and other specialists in your area.

Alabama

University of Alabama at Birmingham
Alzheimer's Disease Center
1720 7th Ave. S., Sparks Center 454
Birmingham AL 35294-0017
Information: (205) 934-2178
Website: http://main.uab.edu/show.asp?durki=11627

Arizona

Sun Health Research Institute
Arizona Alzheimer's Disease Center
1111 East McDowell Rd.
Phoenix AZ 85006
Information: (602) 239-6999
Website: http://mathpost.la.asu.edu/~sampath/index_extA.html

Arkansas

University of Arkansas for Medical Sciences
Alzheimer's Disease Center
4301 W. Markham, Slot 811
Little Rock AR 72205
Information: (501) 603-1294
Website: http://alzheimer.uams.edu

California

Stanford University
Stanford/VA Alzheimer's Disease Research Center
3801 Miranda Ave. (151Y)
Palo Alto CA 94304
Information: (650) 493-5000, ext. 65654
Website: www.stanford.edu/~yesavage/ACRC.html

University of California, Davis
Alzheimer's Disease Center
4860 Y St., Ste. 3700
Sacramento CA 95817
Information: (916) 734-5496
Website: http://alzheimer.ucdavis.edu

University of California, Irvine
Alzheimer's Disease Center
1113 Gillespie Neuroscience Research Facility
Irvine CA 92697
Information: (949) 824-5847
Website: http://alz.uci.edu

University of California, Los Angeles
UCLA Alzheimer's Disease Center
710 Westwood Plaza
Los Angeles CA 90095-1769
Information: (310) 206-5238
Website: www.adc.ucla.edu

University of California, San Diego
San Diego School of Medicine
9500 Gilman Dr.
La Jolla CA 92093-0624
Information: (858) 622-5800
Website: http://adrc.ucsd.edu

University of Southern California
Ethel Percy Andrus Gerontology Center
University Park, MC-0191
3715 McClintock Ave.
Los Angeles CA 90089-0191
Information: (213) 740-7777
Website: www.usc.edu/dept/gero/ADRC

Georgia

Emory University
Emory Alzheimer's Disease Center
1841 Clifton Rd. N.E.
Atlanta GA 30329
Information: (404) 728-6950
Website: www.emory.edu/WHSC/MED/ADC

Illinois

Rush Presbyterian-St. Lukes Medical Center
Rush Alzheimer's Disease Center
1645 West Jackson Blvd., Ste. 675
Chicago IL 60612
Information: (312) 942-4463
Website: www.rush.edu/patients/radc

Northwestern University
Northwestern Alzheimer's Disease Center
675 N. St. Clair, 20th Fl., Ste.100
Chicago IL 60611
Information: (312) 695-9627
Website: www.brain.nwu.edu

Indiana

Indiana University
Indiana Alzheimer's Disease Center, Indiana University
          School of Medicine
635 Barnhill Dr.
Indianapolis IN 46202-5120
Information: (317) 278-2030
Website: http://iadc.iupui.edu

Kentucky

University of Kentucky
Sanders-Brown Center on Aging
800 South Lime St.
Lexington KY 40536-0230
Information: (606) 257-1412
Website: www.coa.uky.edu

Maryland

The Johns Hopkins Medical Institutions
The Johns Hopkins University School of Medicine
720 Rutland Ave.
Baltimore MD 21205-2196
Information: (410) 955-5568
Website: www.alzresearch.org

Massachusetts

Boston University
Boston University Alzheimer's Disease Center
Geriatric Research, Education, and Clinical Center (182B)
Bedford VA Medical Center
200 Springs Rd.
Bedford MA 01730
Information: (617) 687-3167
Website: www.xfaux.com/Alzheimer

Harvard Medical School/Massachusetts General Hospital
Massachusetts Alzheimer's Disease Research Center
WAC 830, 15 Parkman St.
Boston MA 02114
Information: (617) 726-3987
Website: www.madrc.org

Michigan

University of Michigan
Michigan Alzheimer's Disease Research Center
1914 Taubman St.
Ann Arbor MI 48109
Information: (734) 764-2190
Website: www.med.umich.edu/madrc/MADRC.html

Minnesota

Mayo Clinic
Mayo Alzheimer's Disease Center
200 First St. S.W.
Rochester MN 55905
Information: (507) 284-1324
Website: www.mayo.edu/research/alzheimers_center

Missouri

Washington University
Alzheimer's Disease Research Center
Washington University School of Medicine
4488 Forest Park Ave., Ste. 130
St. Louis MO 63108-2293
Information: (314) 286-2881
Website: http://alzheimer.wustl.edu/adrc2/default.htm

New York

Columbia University
Taub Institute for Research on Alzheimer's Disease
630 West 168th St.
New York NY 10032
Information: (212) 305-3300
Website: http://pathology.cpmc.columbia.edu/taub/

Mount Sinai School of Medicine/Bronx VA Medical Center
Mount Sinai Medical Center
1 Gustave L. Levy Pl., Box 1230
New York NY 10029-6574
Information: (212) 241-8329
Website: www.mssm.edu/psychiatry/adrc.shtml

New York University
New York University Medical Center
Silberstein Aging and Dementia Research Center
550 First Ave.
New York NY 10016
Information: (212) 263-8088
Website: http://aging.med.nyu.edu

University of Rochester

University of Rochester Medical Center
Alzheimer's Disease Center
601 Elmwood Ave, Box 603
Rochester NY 14642
Information: (716) 275-2581
Website: www.urmc.rochester.edu/adc/index.html

North Carolina

Duke University

Bryan Alzheimer's Disease Research Center
932 Morreene Rd.
Durham NC 27705
Information: (866) 444-2372
Website: http://adrc.mc.duke.edu/

Ohio

Case Western Reserve University

University Memory and Aging Center
12200 Fairhill Rd.
Cleveland OH 44120
Information: (216) 844-6326
Website: www.ohioalzcenter.org/

Oregon

Oregon Health Sciences University

Oregon Aging and Alzheimer's Disease Center
3181 S. W. Sam Jackson Park Rd.
Portland OR 97201
Information: (503) 494-6976
Website: www.ohsu.edu/som-alzheimers

Pennsylvania

University of Pennsylvania

Alzheimer's Disease Center
Third Floor Maloney Building
3600 Spruce St.
Philadelphia PA 19104
Information: (215) 662-4708
Website: www.uphs.upenn.edu/ADC/

University of Pittsburgh
Alzheimer's Disease Research Center
Montefiore University Hospital, 4 West
200 Lothrop St.
Pittsburgh PA 15213
Information: (412) 692-2700
Website: www.adrc.pitt.edu

Texas

Baylor College of Medicine
Alzheimer's Disease Research Center
6550 Fannin St.
Smith Tower, Ste. 101
Houston TX 77030
Information: (713) 798-6660
Website: www.bcm.tmc.edu/neurol/struct/adrc/adrc1.html

Washington

University of Washington
Alzheimer's Disease Research Center
1660 S. Columbian Way
Seattle WA 98108
Information: (800) 317-5382
Website: http://depts.washington.edu/adrcweb

Print and Video Resources

These recommended books, pamphlets, and educational videotapes are organized according to the chapter headings found in this book. For additional information found on the World Wide Web, see the recommended sites in the Internet Resources.

Chapter 1: The Need for an Accurate Diagnosis

Early Alzheimer's Disease: Patient and Family Guide, Consumer Version, Clinical Practice Guideline Number 19. Rockville, MD: U.S. Department of Health and Human Services, Agency for Health Care Research and Quality (AHRQ), Publication No. 96-0704, 1996. Call the AHRQ Clearinghouse at (800) 358-9295. Also available on-line at: www.ahrq.gov/clinic/alzcons.htm

Dementia Identification and Assessment: Guidelines for Primary Care Practitioners. Washington, DC: Veterans Health Administration, 1997. Available free from: National Center for Cost Containment, U.S. Department of Veteran Affairs, 5000 W. National Ave., Milwaukee WI 53295. Call (414) 384-2000, ext. 2365.

Green R. C. *Diagnosis and Management of Alzheimer's Disease and Other Dementias*. West Islip, NY: Professional Communications, Inc. 2001.

McKhann, G. M., and M. Albert. *Keep Your Brain Young: The Complete Guide to Physical and Emotional Health and Longevity*. New York: John Wiley & Sons, 2002.

Chapter 2: Symptoms of the Early Stages of Alzheimer's Disease

American Health Assistance Foundation. *Honest Answers for the Recently Diagnosed Alzheimer's Patient*. Rockville, MD: American Health Assistance Foundation, 1998. A 43-page booklet for people in the early stages of AD. Call (800) 437-2423.

California Council of the Alzheimer's Association. *Working with Your Doctor When You Suspect Memory Problems*. Los Angeles, CA: California Council of the Alzheimer's Association, 2001. An 18-page booklet about communicating with your physician. Call (916) 447-2731; also available on-line at: www.caalz.org/HKEnglishBooklet.pdf

Davies, H. D., and M. P. Jensen. *Alzheimer's: The Answers You Need*. Forest Knolls, CA: Elder Books, 1998. This book provides answers to over one hundred commonly asked questions; written specifically for persons in the early stages of AD. Call (800) 909-2673.

Gray-Davidson, F. *Alzheimer's Disease: Frequently Asked Questions*. Los Angeles, CA: Lowell House, 1998.

Just For You. Toronto, Canada: Alzheimer Society of Canada, 1995. A ten-page booklet written for people with AD. Call (416) 925-3552.

Molloy, D. W., and J. P. Caldwell. *Alzheimer's Disease: Everything You Need to Know*. Buffalo, NY: Firefly Books, 1998.

Chapter 3: Risk Factors for Developing Alzheimer's Disease

Aisen, P. S., D. B. Marin, and K.L. Davis, eds. *Alzheimer's Disease: Questions and Answers*, 2nd edition. Coral Gables, FL: Merit Publishing International, 1999.

Alzheimer's Disease Progress Report, 2000. Bethesda, MD: National Institutes of Health, National Institute on Aging, Alzheimer's Disease Advisory Panel, 2001. Also available online at: www.alzheimers.org/pubs/prog00.htm

Gillick, M. R. *Tangled Minds: Understanding Alzheimer's Disease and Other Dementias*. New York: Dutton, 1998.

Shenk, D. *The Forgetting: Alzheimer's: Portrait of an Epidemic*. New York: Doubleday, 2001.

Tanzi R. E., and A. B. Parson. *Decoding Darkness: The Search for the Genetic Causes of Alzheimer's Disease*. Cambridge, MA: Perseus Publishing, 2001.

Chapter 4: Progress in Treatment and Prevention of Alzheimer's Disease

Getz, K., and D. Borfitz. *Informed Consent: The Consumer's Guide to the Risks and Benefits of Volunteering for Clinical Trials*. Boston, MA: Thomson/Centerwatch, 2002.

The Alzheimer's Disease Education and Referral Center (ADEAR) publishes *Connections*, a quarterly newsletter sponsored by the U.S. National Institute on Aging that includes updates on research initiatives. Available free from: ADEAR, PO Box 8250, Silver Spring MD 20907-8250. Call (800) 438-4380.

The Alzheimer's Association publishes fact sheets on drugs undergoing testing at research centers and clinics throughout the United States. To obtain fact sheets call (800) 272-3900 or (312) 335-8700.

The National Center for Complementary and Alternative Medicine, a division of the U.S. government's National Institutes of Health, publishes a variety of fact sheets on complementary and alternative medical practices. Call (888) 644-6226.

Small, G. *The Memory Bible: An Innovative Strategy for Keeping Your Brain Young*. New York: Hyperion, 2002.

Chapter 5: What Is It Like to Have Alzheimer's Disease?

Early Alzheimer's: A Forum for Early Stage Dementia Care. (Santa Barbara, CA). A quarterly newsletter for professionals, family members, and individuals in the early stages of AD. Available for $45 annually from: Central Coast Alzheimer's Association, 2024 De La Vina St., Santa Barbara CA 93105. Call (805) 563-0020.

Boden, C. *Who Will I Be When I Die?* East Melbourne, Australia: HarperCollins Religious, 1998.

Braudy, Harris P., ed. *The Person With Alzheimer's Disease: Pathways to Understanding the Experience*. Baltimore, MD: Johns Hopkins University Press, 2002.

Davis, R. *My Journey into Alzheimer's Disease*. Wheaton, IL: Tyndale House Publishers, 1989.

Henderson, C., J. H. Main, R. D. Henderson, and N. Andrews. *Partial View: An Alzheimer's Journal*. Dallas, TX: Southern Methodist University Press, 1998.

McGowin, D. F. *Living in the Labyrinth: A Personal Journey Through the Maze of Alzheimer's*. New York: Delacorte Press, 1993.

Perspectives: A Newsletter for Individuals Diagnosed with Alzheimer's Disease or a Related Disorder. La Jolla, CA. A quarterly publication available for $20 annually through the editor, Lisa Snyder, 9500 Gilman Dr. –0948, La Jolla, CA 92093. Call (858) 622-5800.

Raushi, T. M. *A View from Within: Living with Early Onset Alzheimer's*. Albany, NY: Northeastern Chapter of the Alzheimer's Association, 2001.

Rose, L. *Show Me the Way to Go Home*. Forest Knolls, CA: Elder Books, 1996.

Snyder, L. *Speaking Our Minds: Personal Reflections from Individuals with Alzheimer's Disease*. New York: W. H. Freeman, 1999.

Chapter 6: How Relationships, Roles, and Responsibilities Change

Lustbader, W. *Counting on Kindness: The Dilemmas of Dependency*. New York: The Free Press, 1992.

Lustbader, W., and N. R. Hooyman. *Taking Care of Aging Family Members*. New York: The Free Press, 1994.

Miller S.G. *Unplanned Journey: Understanding the Itinerary*. Wilton, CT: Kaleidoscope Kare, 2000.

Morris, V. *How to Care for Aging Parents*. New York: Workman Publishing, 1996.

Simpson, R., and A. Simpson. *Through the Wilderness of Alzheimer's: A Guide in Two Voices*. Minneapolis, MN: Augsburg Fortress, 1999.

Vanden Bosch, J. *A Thousand Tomorrows: Intimacy, Sexuality and Alzheimer's* (video). Chicago: Terra Nova Films, 1995. Call (800) 779-8491.

Wright, L. K. *Alzheimer's Disease and Marriage*. Newbury Park, CA: Sage Publications, 1993.

Chapter 7: Making Practical Decisions

Family Caregiver Alliance. *Fact Sheet: Driving and Dementia*. Available from Family Caregiver Alliance, 690 Market Street, Ste. 600, San Francisco, CA 94104. Call (415) 434-3388 or go on-line to: www.caregiver.org/factsheets/dementia_driving_national.html

Heath, A. *Long Distance Caregiving: A Survival Guide for Far Away Caregiving*. San Luis Obispo, CA: Impact Publishers, 1993.

National Handbook on Laws and Programs Affecting Senior Citizens.
Chicago: American Bar Association, 1998. Available for $10 from the
Senior Lawyers Division, American Bar Association, 750 N. Lake Shore
Dr., Chicago, IL 60611.

Post, S. G. *The Moral Challenge of Alzheimer's Disease,* 2nd ed. Baltimore,
MD: The Johns Hopkins University Press, 2000.

Tough Issues: Ethical Guidelines of the Alzheimer Society of Canada.
Toronto: Alzheimer Society of Canada, 1998. Available for $15 (U.S.)
from the Task Force on Ethics, Alzheimer Society of Canada, 20 Egling-
ton Ave. W., Ste. 1200, Toronto Ontario M4R 1K8. Call (416) 488-8772
or (800) 616-8816 (toll-free only from within Canada).

Chapter 8: Improving Communication

Bell, V., and D. Troxel. *A Dignified Life: The Best Friends Approach to
Alzheimer's Care.* Deerfield Beach, FL: HCI, Inc. 2002.

Brackey, J. *Creating Moments of Joy for the Person With Alzheimer's or
Dementia: A Journal for Caregivers.* West Lafayette, IN: Purdue University
Press, 2000.

Kitwood, T. *Dementia Reconsidered: The Person Comes First.* Buckingham,
England: Open University Press, 1998. Call (800) 821-8312.

A Part of Daily Life: Alzheimer's Caregivers Simplify Activities and the Home
(video). Washington, DC: American Occupational Therapy Foundation,
1993. May be available through the local chapter of the Alzheimer's
Association or may be purchased or rented through Terra Nova Films.
Call (800) 779-8491.

Rau, M. T. *Coping with Communication Challenges in Alzheimer's Disease.*
San Diego, CA: Singular Publishing Group, 1993.

Starkman, E. M. *Learning to Sit in Silence: A Journal of Caretaking.*
Watsonville, CA: Papier-Mache Press, 1994.

Strauss, C. J. *Talking to Alzheimer's: Simple Ways to Connect When You Visit
with a Family Member or Friend.* Oakland, CA: New Harbinger Publications, 2001.

Chapter 9: Helping a Person with AD to Plan for the Future

Carlin, V. F., and V. E. Greenberg. *Should Mom Live with Us? And Is Happiness Possible if She Does?* New York: Free Press, 1992.

Family Guide for Alzheimer Care in Residential Settings. Chicago, IL:
Alzheimer's Association, 1992.

A Home Away from Home: A Consumer Guide to Board and Care Homes and Assisted Living Facilities. Washington, DC: AARP, 1995.

In Your Hands: The Tools for Preserving Personal Autonomy (video). Chicago, IL: American Bar Association, 1997. Available for purchase or rental through Terra Nova Films. Call (800) 779-8491.

Residential Care: A Guide for Choosing a New Home. Chicago: Alzheimer's Association, 1999.

Strauss, P. J., and N. M. Lederman. *The Elder Law Handbook: A Legal and Financial Survival Guide for Caregivers and Seniors.* New York: Facts on File, 1996.

Tomorrow's Choices: Preparing Now for Future Legal, Financial and Health-care decisions. Washington, DC: AARP, 1992.

White, L., and B. Spencer. *Moving a Relative with Memory Loss.* Santa Rosa, CA: Whisp Publications, 2000.

Chapter 10: Keeping a Person with AD Active and Healthy

Clair, A. A. *Therapeutic Uses of Music with Older Adults.* Baltimore, MD: Health Professions Press, 1996.

Cordrey, C. *Hidden Treasures: Music and Memory Activities for People with Alzheimer's.* Mt. Airy, MD: ElderSong Publications, 1994.

Decker, J. A. *Making the Moments Count: Leisure Activities for Caregiving Relationships.* Baltimore, MD: Johns Hopkins University Press, 1995.

Fitzray, B. J. *Alzheimer's Activities: Hundreds of Activities for Men and Women With Alzheimer's Disease and Related Disorders.* Windsor, CA: Rayve Productions, 2001.

Gwyther, L. P. *You Are One of Us: Successful Clergy/Church Connections to Alzheimer's Families.* Durham, NC: Center for Aging Alzheimer's Family Support Program, Duke University Medical Center, 1995.

Steps to Planning Activities. Chicago: Alzheimer's Association, 1995.

Walker, S. *Keeping Active: A Caregiver's Guide to Activities with the Elderly.* San Luis Obispo, CA: Impact Publishers, 1994.

Information Especially for Children and Teens

Fading Memories: An Adolescent's Guide to Alzheimer's Disease. Available for $5 from the American Health Assistance Program, 15825 Shady Grove Rd., Ste. 140, Rockville MD 20850. Call (800) 437-2423.

Gosselin K. *Allie Learns About Alzheimer's Disease: A Family Story About Love, Patience, and Acceptance.* Plainview, NY: JayJo Books, 2002.

Just for Children and *Just for Teens: Helping You Understand Alzheimer's Disease by the Alzheimer's Association.* Two fact sheets available for free from the Alzheimer's Association, 919 N. Michigan Ave., Ste. 1000, Chicago IL 60611. Call (800) 272-3900 or (312) 335-5796.

McCrea, J. M. *Talking with Children and Teens About Alzheimer's Disease: A Question and Answer Guidebook for Parents, Teachers, and Caregivers.* Pittsburgh, PA: Univ. of Pittsburgh, 1994, seventy-five pages. Available for $15 from Generations Together, University of Pittsburgh, 121 University Pl., Ste. 300, Pittsburgh PA 15260. Call (412) 648-7150.

Someone I Love Has Alzheimer's Disease. The Alzheimer's Association of Eastern Massachusetts. A seventeen-minute video and curriculum guide available for $24.95 from InJoy Productions, 3970 Broadway, Ste. B4, Boulder CO 80304. Call (800) 326-2082.

Through Tara's Eyes: Helping Children Cope with Alzheimer's Disease. Available for $5 from the American Health Assistance Program, 15825 Shady Grove Rd., Ste. 140, Rockville MD 20850. Call (800) 437-2423.

Chapter 11: Self-Renewal for Family and Friends

Barg, G. *The Fearless Caregiver: How to Get the Best for Your Loved One and Still Have a Life of Your Own.* Hendon, VA: Capitol Books, 2001.

Chapman, J. *Journaling for Joy: Writing Your Way to Personal Growth and Freedom.* North Hollywood, CA: Newcastle, 1991.

Ewing, W. *Tears in God's Bottle: Reflections on Alzheimer's Caregiving.* Tucson, AZ: WhiteStone Circle Press, 1999.

Kushner, H. S. *When Bad Things Happen to Good People.* New York: Avon Books, 1981.

Lustbader, W. *A Prescription for Caregivers: Take Care of Yourself* (video). Seattle, WA: Wendy Lustbader, 1997. Available for purchase or rental through Terra Nova Films. Call (800) 779-8491.

Witrogen-McLeod, B. *Caregiving: The Spiritual Journey of Love, Loss, and Renewal.* New York: John Wiley & Sons, 1999.

Chapter 12: Obtaining the Help You May Need

Bridges, B. J. *Therapeutic Caregiving: A Practical Guide for Caregivers of Persons with Alzheimer's and Other Dementia-Causing Diseases.* Mill Creek, WA: BJB Publishing, 1995.

Educational Media Services and L. P. Gwyther. *From Here to Hope: The Stages of Alzheimer's Disease* (video). Durham, NC: Duke University Medical Center, 1998. Call (919) 684-3748.

Mace, N. L., and P. V. Rabins. *The 36-Hour Day: A Family Guide to Caring for Persons with Alzheimer's Disease, Related Dementing Illnesses, and Memory Loss in Later Life,* third ed. Baltimore, MD: Johns Hopkins University Press, 1999.

Mittelman M. S., C. Epstein, and A. Pierzchala. *Counseling the Alzheimer's Caregiver.* Chicago, IL: AMA Press, 2003. Although primarily a resource for professionals, this book covers a variety of practical issues in a very readable fashion. Call (800) 621-8335.

Susik, H. *Hiring Home Caregivers.* San Luis Obispo, CA: Impact Publishers, 1995.

Taxes and Alzheimer's Disease. A series of short publications on a variety of tax issues that are periodically updated. Contact the public policy office of the Alzheimer's Association, 1319 F St. N.W., Ste. 710, Washington DC, 20004. Call (202) 393-7737.

Chapter 13: Voices of Experience

Bryan, J., ed. *Love Is Ageless: Stories About Alzheimer's Disease,* second ed. Felton, CA: Lampico Creek Press, 2002.

Dyer, J. *In a Tangled Wood: An Alzheimer's Journey.* Dallas, TX: Southern Methodist University Press, 1996.

Haisman, P. *Alzheimer's Disease: Caregivers Speak Out.* Fort Myers, FL: Chippendale House Publishers, 1998.

Mathiasen, P. *An Ocean of Time: Alzheimer's Tales of Hope and Forgetting.* New York: Scribner, 1997.

Mitchell, M. *Dancing on Quicksand: A Gift of Friendship in the Age of Alzheimer's.* Boulder, CO: Johnson Books, 2002.

Young, E. P. *Between Two Worlds: Special Moments of Alzheimer's & Dementia.* Amherst, NY: Prometheus Books, 1999.

Internet Resources

This section contains information about Internet websites and e-mail groups devoted to Alzheimer's disease, related disorders, and other topics of interest.

The 1990s will be remembered as the decade in which people first became electronically linked on a massive scale through a network of computer networks known as the Internet. Tens of millions of people worldwide now have quick and easy access to one another. Electronic messages, also known as e-mail, can be sent and received across the globe, enabling almost instantaneous communication. The medium of the Internet promises to be the quickest, easiest, and least expensive means to learn about anything, including AD.

Billions of pages of information on virtually any topic are available through the fastest growing part of the Internet known as the World Wide Web. The Web consists of text, graphics, and audio and video information supplied by individuals and organizations that create sites that people can visit with the aid of a computer, a telephone line or cable, and a software program called a browser. There are dozens of sites devoted exclusively to AD care, education, and research that offer an amazing amount of information about the disease. Most of these sites are updated regularly and provide links to related sites on the Web. Yet there are pitfalls, too. The facts and opinions posted on websites can be informative at best, misleading at worst. The quality of information ranges from excellent to very poor, so care is needed in sorting out truth from fiction. It is best to find out who the authors or the organizations sponsoring a website are to determine the reliability and currency of its information.

At present, there is no good way to evaluate the content of sites, although some health-care providers are developing guidelines, standards, and "seals of approval" to assist consumers. In the meantime, you will need to be careful in choosing which sites are most reliable.

The Internet also enables individuals to electronically communicate with other individuals or groups who share similar interests in so-called discussion groups, bulletin boards, and chat rooms. The quality of information shared on-line depends entirely upon the individuals who are participating, although sometimes a group leader or sponsor is available to offer limited oversight. Information is typically exchanged informally and anecdotally, so facts always need to be checked out.

Listed below are some selected Internet resources that have proven to be both trustworthy and informative.

Alzheimer's Discussion Group

This is an e-mail group sponsored by the Alzheimer's Disease Research Center at Washington University in St. Louis at (314) 362-2882. It is open to anyone and subscription is free. There are thousands of subscribers worldwide, generating at least fifty messages daily. To subscribe, send an e-mail message to:

majordomo@wubios.wustl.edu

and in the body of the message, type the following:

subscribe alzheimer-digest

Within hours you should receive a confirmation message that tells you how to complete the simple process. If you wish to receive individual messages from this group instead of receiving them bundled into a daily digest, follow the same instructions but type "subscribe alzheimer" only.

Alzheimer's Bulletin Boards and Chat Rooms

Commercial on-line services such as Prodigy Internet and America Online offer an array of bulletin boards and chat rooms devoted to specific medical problems, including Alzheimer's disease. Check with each service.

Websites About Alzheimer's Disease

All of the federally funded AD centers in the United States operate websites; their names and Internet addresses are listed in the first section of the Resources. Other excellent websites are given below, and are, in turn, linked to other sites of interest.

The Alzheimer's Disease Education and Referral Center

www.alzheimers.org

(800) 438-4380

This clearinghouse is funded by The National Institute on Aging, a U.S. government agency based in Bethesda, Maryland. A Combined Health Information Database (CHID) at this site contains references to and abstracts of more than 7,000 educational materials on AD. Information about drugs in testing is also available at this site. Informative pamphlets, research reports, and the Center's newsletters can be viewed and downloaded.

The Alzheimer's Association

www.alz.org

(800) 272-3900

(312) 335-8700

This voluntary health organization based in Chicago coordinates the efforts of over a hundred chapters in the United States, promotes changes in public policy, and funds research. This site provides much helpful information and can link you to local chapters, many of which operate their own websites. The Association's numerous publications and reading lists on over two dozen topics of interest can be found at this site.

Alzheimer Society of Canada

www.alzheimer.ca

(800) 616-8816 (toll-free only from within Canada)

(414) 488-8722

This voluntary health organization based in Toronto coordinates the efforts of the provincial societies throughout Canada, promotes policy changes, and funds research. The site offers information about AD in both English and French.

Alzheimer's Disease International
www.alz.co.uk
This is an international association based in London with more than sixty member countries with Alzheimer's associations. This site offers links to many of these member countries and contains useful information on the worldwide scope of AD.

Alzheimer Europe
www.alzheimer-europe.org
This site is maintained by the organization serving European countries and therefore has a lot of information in many languages, including English, French, German, Spanish, Dutch, Portuguese, Swedish, Danish, and Finnish.

Alzheimer Web
www.alzweb.org
This was one of the first sites devoted to AD and continues to provide current information about medical advances and information about caring for someone with the disease.

Alzheimer's Research Forum
www.alzforum.org
Although this site is mainly for researchers, it posts news articles, runs forums, and lists resources that may be of general interest to everyone.

Dementia Advocacy and Support Network
www.dasninternational.org
This site was established by a small but growing organization of people with AD and other dementias. It serves as a forum to promote respect and dignity for persons with dementia and to exchange information. It also provides a link to an electronic support group for people with dementia.

Dementia Web
http://dementia.ion.ucl.ac.uk
This site is sponsored by the Dementia Research Group, comprised of a number of scientists and health-care professionals in London. It contains information, advice, and research findings about AD and has a special section about the rare form of the disease affecting middle-aged people.

Doctor's Guide to Alzheimer's Disease Information and Resources
www.pslgroup.com/alzheimer.htm
The information available on this site is geared to practicing physicians but clearly may be of interest to others. You may want to recommend this site to your physician.

Medline Plus
www.nlm.nih.gov/medlineplus/alzheimersdisease.html
A service of the U.S. National Library of Medicine, the latest research findings on AD are posted here.

National Institute of Neurological Disorders and Stroke
www.ninds.nih.gov/health_and_medical/disorders/alzheimersdisease_doc. htm
Part of the U.S. National Institutes of Health, this site offers numerous fact sheets on AD and other dementias.

Websites on Related Dementias

Other Dementias
www.zarcrom.com/users/alzheimers/odem/index1.html
This site is devoted to the wide variety of dementias other than Alzheimer's disease and includes links to many of the sites noted below as well as several others.

Parkinson's Disease

U.S. National Institutes of Health Parkinson's Disease Information Page
www.ninds.nih.gov/health_and_medical/disorders/parkinsons_disease.htm

The Parkinson's Web, Harvard University
http://pdweb.mgh.harvard.edu

National Parkinson Foundation, Inc.
www.parkinson.org
(800) 327-4545

American Parkinson's Disease Association, Inc.
www.apdaparkinson.com
(800) 223-2732

Lewy Body Disease
www.ccc.nottingham.ac.uk/~mpzjlowe/lewy/lewyhome.html
This site offers comprehensive information on Lewy body disease or dementia with Lewy bodies, including abstracts of numerous scientific papers on this form of dementia. This form of dementia can be character-ized as a combination of both AD and Parkinson's disease and often includes psychiatric features such as hallucinations and delusions.

Pick's Disease
This is also a rare form of dementia in which behavioral or personality

changes are first observed, followed by memory loss and other cognitive impairments.

The Pick's Disease Support Group
www.pdsg.org.uk
E-mail discussion group: http://groups.yahoo.com/group/picks-support/

Creutzfeldt-Jakob Disease
This is a rare form of dementia that is usually rapidly progressive and mainly affects memory and motor functions.

CJD Voice
www.cjdvoice.org

The Creutzfeldt-Jakob Foundation
http://members.aol.com/crjakob/intro.html

Primary Progressive Aphasia
This is another rare brain disorder first marked by the gradual loss of speech and, in most cases, eventual memory impairment.

Primary Progressive Aphasia Newsletter
www.brain.nwu.edu/ppa/

Huntington's Disease
This is a rare disorder due to a genetic mutation manifested by progressive motor and memory impairments occurring before middle age.

The Huntington's Disease Society of America
www.hdsa.org
(800) 345-HDSA

International Huntington Association
www.huntington-assoc.com

Down's Syndrome and Alzheimer's Disease
Down's syndrome is a form of mental retardation associated with a genetic mutation. Many people with this syndrome develop AD in middle age.

The Arc
www.TheArc.org/misc/alzbk.html

Other Websites of Interest

U. S. Government Sites

National Center for Complementary and Alternative Medicine
http://nccam.nih.gov
(888) 644-6226

Comprehensive descriptions about types of alternative medicine, as well as research projects on alternative medicine currently funded by the U.S. government's chief medical research agency, the National Institutes of Health, are given on this site.

Healthfinder
www.healthfinder.gov
A searchable list of dozens of health-related sources of information.

The Food and Drug Administration
www.fda.gov
This is the U.S. government agency responsible for overseeing the safety and effectiveness of all foods and drugs sold in the United States.

The Administration on Aging
www.aoa.dhhs.gov/aoa/pages/jpostlst.html
This site offers links to hundreds of resources on age-related issues.

Social Security Administration
www.ssa.gov
(800) 772-1234
This agency is responsible for tax-funded retirement and disability programs.

Medicare
www.medicare.gov
(800) MEDICARE
This site is devoted to consumer information about all aspects of this major insurance program for elderly and disabled Americans administered by the Centers for Medicare and Medicaid Services.

Eldercare Locator
www.eldercare.gov
(800) 677-1116
This is a nationwide database, administered by the National Association of Area Agencies on Aging, that offers lists of local services for older people and their families.

Legal and Financial Planning

National Senior Citizens Law Center
www.nsclc.org
(202) 289-6796 Washington, D.C. office
(213) 639-0930 Los Angeles office
This is a nonprofit group that advocates for the legal rights of older Americans.

National Academy of Elder Law Attorneys, Inc.

www.naela.org

(520) 881-4005

This nonprofit organization assists attorneys, bar organizations, and others who work with older people and their families.

Financial Planning Association

www.fpanet.org

(800) 647-6340

This is a professional association of more than 15,000 financial planners nationwide.

Medicine and Health Issues

Clinical Trials

www.ClinicalTrials.gov

The U.S. National Institutes of Health developed this site to provide individuals, family members, and members of the public with current information about clinical research studies. At any given time, more than two dozen clinical trials for AD drugs are listed as well as sites where the studies are being conducted throughout the United States.

Pharmaceutical Research and Manufacturers of America

www.phrma.org

(800) 762-4636

This site includes the "Directory of Prescription Drug Patient Assistance Programs."

Mayo Clinic's Health Oasis

www.mayoclinic.com/findinformation/diseasesandconditions/index.cfm

You'll find a wealth of information about health matters, including AD, provided by the Mayo Clinic based in Rochester, Minnesota.

Housing Options

American Association of Homes and Services for the Aging

www.aahsa.org

(202) 783-2242

A nonprofit organization representing more than five thousand nursing homes, retirement communities, assisted-living facilities, senior housing developments, and community agencies.

Assisted Living Federation of America

www.alfa.org

(703) 691-8100

A nonprofit organization representing assisted-living facilities throughout the United States.

American Health Care Association
www.ahca.org
(202) 842-4444
A federation of organizations representing long-term-care providers.

Senior Alternatives
www.senioralternatives.com
A nationwide directory of housing options and other services for older people.

Family Support

National Family Caregivers Association
www.nfcacares.org
(800) 535-3198
A nonprofit educational and advocacy organization in support of families that provide care to loved ones of all ages.

National Alliance for Caregiving
www.caregiving.org
A nonprofit joint venture of numerous organizations to support family caregivers of the elderly and the professionals who serve them. This site contains reports, products, and helpful tips.

Family Caregiver Alliance
www.caregiver.org
(415) 434-3388
This nonprofit organization serves residents of California who care for brain-impaired adults; the site has lots of information useful to all those caring for persons with AD.

National Association of Professional Geriatric Care Managers
www.caremanager.org
(520) 881-8008
This nonprofit organization of more than one thousand professionals throughout the United States assists families in caring for older adults and disabled persons on a fee-for-service basis.

Faith in Action
www.fiavolunteers.org
(877) 324-8411
This is an interfaith volunteer program of The Robert Wood Johnson Foundation with nearly 1,200 programs throughout the United States. It works to improve the lives of people of all ages and their families coping with long-term illnesses or disabilities.

Shepherd's Centers of America
www.shepherdcenters.org
(800) 547-7073
(816) 960-2022
This interfaith, nonprofit organization coordinates nearly 100 independent centers throughout the United States with volunteer programs that help keep older people as independent as possible and assist family caregivers.

Index

. . . .